HIPPOLITE AMADI

BORN TO LIVE NOT TO DIE

ONE MAN'S BATTLE TO OVERCOME CORRUPTION
AND SAVE THE LIVES OF NIGERIAN BABIES

Mereo Books

Mereo Books 2nd Floor, 6-8 Dyer Street,
Cirencester, Gloucestershire, GL7 2PF

An imprint of Memoirs Book Ltd. www.mereobooks.com

Born to live, not to die: 978-1-86151-952-8

First published in Great Britain in 2020
by Mereo Books, an imprint of Memoirs Books Ltd.

The address for Memoirs Books Ltd. can be
found at www.memoirspublishing.com

Memoirs Books Ltd. Reg. No. 7834348

Typeset in 10/15pt Sabon
by Wiltshire Associates Ltd.
Printed and bound in Great Britain

PREFACE

✦✦✦✦✦✦✦

In this drama which has been my life and career, I have written about the events that unfolded based on my own perception and interpretation. It is understandable that my impressions could be different from what the people in my story intended to achieve with their behaviour, whether positive or negative. Every day, our good and bad utterances and our body language amount to pages that could be put into a book by someone observing the events.

We may be able to decide the character we wish to represent and be careful to portray this by our actions in daily living. How wonderful it would feel if someone's input in a narrative led to great outcomes as the drama of this story unfolds. This becomes a positive character to emulate in the midst of other less positive ones. I challenge young people from poorer countries who are studying in developed countries to remain focused, patient with their supervisors and be excellent team players in their research groups, as this way happier stories could be told in the places where sad ones had been taking centre stage.

I wish to stress that prior to the unfolding of this life drama, there was nothing so special about me as a person to make anyone want to assist me or fight for my promotion; absolutely nothing! Having been rejected, I miraculously defied expectations to become a pillar in the defence of neonatal life.

I strictly ensured that prior to publication of this book, no one – including any of my immediate and extended family members – had any opportunity of reading this manuscript to influence or modify whatever I have written or my opinions as documented. Hence, I am fully responsible and should be held solely accountable for the content of this book.

Hippolite Amadi

To my wife, Iphii and my children –
Ugo, Jimara, Zina, Cherie & Matie

(for all they had to endure as I did this work)

CONTENTS

✦✦✦✦✦✦✦

FOREWORD

✦✦✦✦✦✦✦

Born to live, not to die is a unique book. Although its theme is a popular one, the manner of presentation is refreshingly different. Neonatal mortality in Nigeria and Africa is not particularly new, but one would think that whoever would write on it would be an obstetrician or a midwife. The author of this book is neither. It is also not a book written for professionals only. It is a story written for the lay public and will bring to their consciousness what truly concerns them. It tells the story of the efforts of a Nigerian medical engineer to eliminate the needless deaths of neonates in Nigeria.

This is what makes the story of Professor Hippolite Amadi unique: its authorship, its audience and manner of address. The medical personnel in Nigeria questioned his authority to speak for the neonate, not being primarily a medical doctor. They also questioned his credentials, not having attended any university in England or America. The admin staff had a different type of grouse: Hippolite would not grease their palms. In his attempt to overcome these odds, Hippolite had to move to England to enhance his authority, introduce to Nigeria the benefit of multidisciplinary approach in keeping neonates alive and confront the greed of some medical personnel who were exploiting the corruption in hospitals.

Undoubtedly, neonates still die in Nigeria, multidisciplinary cooperation is not yet fully accepted and corruption still exists in the supply and maintenance of incubators and neonatal devices. However, Hippolite's achievements and the manner of securing them are not only outstanding but so unique that writing this book becomes the best way of moving the battle to save neonates to its next stage. That next stage is to take the battle from the trenches and hidden places into the open fields to the doorstep of the ignorant parent, the legislature, the campaigner for the rights of the new-born baby, the religious organisations and young people.

Hippolite's travails are myriad: rejection of his various incubators tailor-made for the Nigerian health facility, dislike for his strong Christian convictions and distrust of his patriotism. This book does not just tell us how he overcame them but serves as a template for those who intend to overcome similar problems in other fields of endeavour. We also read of the heroic support he received from home and abroad: his university and church in England and his friends and associates in Nigeria. In summary, this book is about a typical 'war and triumph' story. There were plights and perils faced but surmounted. It is however a continuing battle that concerns all, whether as parent or simply someone who cares for children.

Hippolite has thus provided all Nigerians and the citizens of the world with an opportunity to participate in the battle to save the Nigerian and African neonate. He has written the book in a simple way, avoiding discouraging technical jargon. I truly hope that enlistment to this battle will begin with reading the book and taking decisive action in bringing to light the needless deaths of the poor defenceless neonates who are born to live and not to die.

OLUWEMIMO OGUNDE SAN
Formerly Attorney-General, Ogun State, Nigeria

INTRODUCTION

✦✦✦✦✦✦✦

I could not stop wondering about the misfortunes of newborn babies in Africa. Even when I tried to shrug the problem off, it was still there clouding my mind. Why was Africa so backward in development? Why was it so backward in creating its own solutions to solve its own peculiar needs?

I went to bed thinking of Africa's true technological emancipation, which has eluded many generations across this vast continent. What bothered me most was not Africa's extreme poverty only, I was much more bothered that these thoughts refused to leave my mind; I went to bed thinking about Africa and woke up with the same thoughts. Something had to be wrong somewhere.

In this day and age, I do not want to be part of an Africa that constantly begs the Western world for technological and medical aids and help, constantly feels inferior on the global stage and is constantly made to believe that her people were created to be dependent on the Western countries. I do not want to belong to an Africa that maintains a slavish mentality towards the lighter-skinned people in the West and is intimidated into believing that it is unable to create science and technology. Nor do I want to belong to a land that constantly supports the lie that Africans are unable to produce the technologies needed for their ever-growing needs.

I believed that modern Africa should consciously work for her technological and commercial independence, not demand financial aid from people who gave them pennies with one hand and took them away with the other. I wanted Africa to stop begging for a slice of the foreign cake. I believed the Africa of today should rather ask to be shown how to bake a cake, so as to produce appropriate cultural and climate-compatible versions, for no one should understand Africa better than the Africans. I believed the Africa of today should aim to produce a new breed of scientists capable of creating local content and useful technologies – technologies that would address Africa's specific needs. Africans should patronise their home-made technologies whilst encouraging their continuous development and growth.

Such thoughts, visions and dreams motivated a bold move which would demonstrate the impact of African-powered modern technology, inspired by an African-specific healthcare need. In my medical adventures I made enemies, broke barriers, pushed boundaries, carried out dangerous manoeuvres, made and destroyed friendships, all in the attempt to wage war against a high neonatal mortality rate in the nation of Nigeria. The vision was crazy and the moves were radical, but I was unstoppable.

CHAPTER 1

THE SEEDS OF AN IDEA

✦✦✦✦✦✦✦

In June 1987, three years before the inception of the United Nations Millennium Development Goals (MDG) programme in Nigeria, as a young engineering student at Anambra State University of Technology (ASUTECH), I visited the city of Port Harcourt in southern Nigeria. The iconic Ebony Hospitals Limited was in the Rumola area of the garden city of Port Harcourt. In the hospital's Medical Diagnostic Laboratory, Austin, a medical laboratory scientist, was operating his manually-operated, two-bucket centrifuge and sweating profusely as he laboured with the spinning mechanism to sediment a set of blood samples.

Then a fourth-year mechanical engineering student, I

watched in amazement and wondered why this procedure could not be carried out differently. 'What is this machine called and why must you spend such a long time and so much energy doing this one action when electricity could be harnessed to spin this for you?' I asked. 'That would release you to do other things, you know.' I pulled a face in bewilderment.

'This machine is called a centrifuge,' said Austin. 'It is used to sediment particles of a solution according to their respective particulate weights. It does this by generating centrifugal forces that act on the fluid when the test-tube is vigorously spun as you saw me do. Electric centrifuges exist, but the imported machine is very expensive and hardly affordable.'

With a deep sense of concern and wonder, I said, 'Okay, but this doesn't look so complicated that a company in this country couldn't manufacture it, does it?'

Austin was uncomfortable at hearing such a bold question from a student who was so much younger than him. Leaning forward as if to whisper a secret, he challenged me that if I could bring such technology to Nigeria I would have distinguished myself so greatly that it would guarantee me a great future.

'Did you just say great future?' I asked, wondering if this was as serious as Austin was making it sound.

'Great future, yes I really mean that,' said Austin. 'This is the first machine any serious medical laboratory must have, yet every single one in this country has been imported. Can you imagine the impact you would make, given the size of Nigeria?'

Austin reached for a small plastic jar on his desk. The jar was filled with roasted peanuts. He removed his gloves and took a handful. 'I love peanuts,' he said, holding out the jar to offer me some nuts. 'Yes I really mean it – great future, huge national impact.'

Austin's words kept reverberating in my mind all through that day and the days following. This simple event marked the beginning of a technological storm that would change the vision of a young engineering student forever and boldly challenge Nigeria to look inwards for solutions that would address one of her most challenging medical technology needs – innovating appropriate devices and procedures for the reduction of high neonatal mortality rate (NNMR).

There was only six months to go before I would be required by the University to propose my final year degree project. This was the mandatory design and production of an engineering system at the University. The challenge from Austin prompted me to initiate a literature search to enable me to fully understand the principles of centrifugal forces as harnessed in medical devices. Soon I proposed the design and production of an automatic medical laboratory centrifuge. This was approved, and it was to be supervised by one of Nigeria's finest professors of mechanical engineering at Asutech, Professor Ofodile.

The subsequent academic defence of the completed project was spectacularly advertised by the Department of Mechanical/Production Engineering during the 1988 cohort exams. It was an 'A' rated project output which the University showcased during internal and external exhibitions in the years that followed. However, none of the professors were smart enough to advise the university concerning the possibilities of a 'spin-off' company arising from such successful projects. This kind of failure to convert raw ideas has remained the downfall of African technology to the present day.

I left the university that same year as the top graduating student from my class. Austin's words remained fresh in my mind during the design stage of the project. Upon approval for production of the system to begin, I said to my supervisor, 'Professor, it is my intention to produce three prototypes of this system'.

'No, there is no need for that. Any particular reason?' asked Professor Ofodile.

'Yes sir, I will need to carry out some independent performance analyses of the prototype at the Port Harcourt hospital where I first heard of laboratory centrifuge,' I replied. At that time I had never seen an electrically-powered centrifuge. I only drew inspiration from the manually-operated version at Ebony Hospital.

'Okay, that won't be a problem provided your dad is willing to fund the huge cost of the workshop materials that will be required,' said the supervisor. My uncle (Izume), whom I later called 'Papa,' was a visionary consultant hand surgeon trained at the great University of Heidelberg in Germany. Papa passionately sought the industrialisation of Africa and often challenged me that the continent's future relied on the emergence of would-be 'creative thinkers'. Papa and my adorable elder brother Chukwuebuka ('Chubuks') did not hesitate to support me with the funding for the production of the prototypes after I enthusiastically explained how I hoped to progress with my new invention. Papa and Professor Ofodile were both very proud of me, and would later become good friends.

One of the systems was sent off to Ebony Hospital, where it satisfactorily completed all clinical tests. The hospital later paid off the cost of two thousand Nigerian naira (₦2,000) and kept the system for use at its laboratory; thus Ebony Hospital became the first medical institution ever to apply any medical product from this would-be great African thinker, early in 1988. The director of the hospital, Dr Centy, was particularly proud of this, especially as his hometown of origin was the same village as mine. The ₦2,000 'first fruit' was carefully put in the bank as I set off for my mandatory post-graduation one year paramilitary service in Baguda State in the north-west of Nigeria.

The hopes and aspirations of thousands of budding young African scientists are often dashed as soon as they show signs of their potential. They are being destroyed daily by gangs of government officials in similar circumstances as those I experienced in the city of Baguda. The Nigerian National Youth Service Corps (NYSC) was the dream of every young Nigerian studying at institutions of higher learning. It was a programme that showcased the great strengths of the future Nigeria, reassuring hopes through the great army of young graduates that congregated yearly for this service. It was a national honour to appear in the official NYSC regalia and every 'Youth Corper' was treated with respect as a 'Federal government special child'.

Youth Corps members did a wide range of volunteer community services for their country. They were accordingly rewarded in goodwill and encouragement. The Emir of Baguda, then the Chancellor of the university I had graduated from, was glad to know that I had been posted to serve in his home state. He remembered me winning lots of awards during the last graduation ceremony at Enugu University. He invited me to his palace and encouraged me to pay a visit to the State's Commissioner of Health to demonstrate the laboratory centrifuge he had seen at Enugu earlier in the year.

At the Emir's request, the office of the Commissioner of Health gave me an appointment to meet with the Commissioner, Dr Jusa. The system was demonstrated on the appointed day and the Commissioner seemed pleasantly surprised that a young Nigerian engineer could manufacture such an automatic system with such a high level of precision and finish. He praised my ingenuity to the applause of all present, almost repeating the very words Austin, the scientist, had used two years earlier.

I became excited and began to think seriously about Austin's challenge. Was it possible to form a manufacturing company as a spin-off from this? How great if every young African student could be made to think beyond the university when choosing a degree project! It could also be possible, even in Africa, to develop a university project into an industrial product that could impact the entire world.

Unfortunately, Africa did not seem to have the right calibre of professors to encourage young science students. Young people could invest all their youthful energies in spin-off industries if well-guided by well-meaning academics, politicians and industrialists. These were lacking, unfortunately. However, it was important to challenge young people to think positively, with or without these adults around them who were so lacking in vision.

I wondered what more I could take out of my meeting with

the Commissioner. But just as I was about to thank him for the audience, he made an offer that blew me away.

'I am very excited about this invention and I think my Ministry has to take this up to show Nigerian society how fantastic a young Nigerian engineer could be,' he said, to the approval of the small audience that were watching the exhibition. I could not hide my emotion as I replied, 'thank you sir, thank you sir!'

'Given this support, would you be able to start up the production of more units of this system, progressing to different stages of completion to be exhibited for the public, say up to ten units?' asked the Commissioner.

'Yes sir, this is quite possible, sir,' I replied.

'In that case I would like you to come back to my office next week with your proposals and cost implications for further discussion on this matter'.

I was delighted. I hurried off to telephone the good news to my mentor, Professor Ofodile. Having received further advice from the professor, I went on to prepare for my next meeting with Commissioner Jusa. But I had no idea how quickly things could change for the most trivial reasons.

There were a lot of people in the Commissioner's waiting room that morning when I arrived. Dr Jusa and his long entourage did not walk in until I had been waiting for a couple of hours. I never noticed him walk in, as I was studying my write-up. The entire atmosphere was strange to me; the culture of the northern people of Nigeria was still unfamiliar, as I had lived all my life in the east with its completely different culture. I did not guess why there was a sudden movement of people in the room; I only realised that the others had suddenly stood up. So I looked up and there was Dr Jusa looking down at me. I quickly stood, but Dr Jusa ignored my greeting and walked into his office.

I was a total stranger to the Muslim culture of northern Nigeria as I had never been to the north, let alone had any experience of the Islamic culture before my NYSC posting. Well-meaning Nigerians do appreciate the possible culture shocks that Corps members might encounter and are readily prepared to help and not to punish them. Unfortunately I was to be a victim of this cultural clash of Eastern vs Northern Nigeria. This probably led to the dashing of all the hopes Dr Jusa had raised during the earlier meeting. The Commissioner's interest in me suddenly evaporated, simply because he felt I had refused to respect him as others did by standing before his entry. I would not have had any problem standing up if I had known that this was the culture, or seen Dr Jusa walking in. My later suspicion was that an office assistant might have announced his approach to the office in the Hausa language, which I did not understand. There was no way I could have understood what was said, especially as I was studying my script. What a sad situation!

When I was finally called in to see Dr Jusa, he treated me with unbelievable contempt. The formerly excited Commissioner had turned unwelcoming and grumpy. Now away from the watching public, the Commissioner said to me, 'I don't quite remember who you are'. I tried to remind him of the demonstration I had done only the previous week and of the Commissioner's promise and invitation leading to the current appointment. But it was possible that Dr Jusa might not have meant his promise. He either made the promises to impress the few individuals that were present at the time, or broken it as a consequence of not 'respecting' him when he had entered.

So I left Dr Jusa's office with my hopes dashed. Could this be the end of the celebrated invention? I decided to concentrate on my NYSC primary assignment, but I kept wondering how to utilize any other opportunity that might arise later.

CHAPTER 2

AN ENTREPRENEUR IS BORN

✦✦✦✦✦✦✦

Immediately after the completion of my National Youth Service, I returned to the university and completed my Master's degree in Mechanical Engineering Technology & Management. I spent private time in the university workshop to produce three more units of my automatic centrifuge, now referred to as the 'Polite 450 Automatic Laboratory Centrifuge (P450)' for commercial purposes. One unit was happily purchased by the Medical Laboratory Unit of Grand Hospital Uyo, owned by my uncle. Many in my extended family were happy for me and wanted to find ways of encouraging me to make a good start in life. Auntie Beatty, a senior staff member at the Imo Blood Bank, broke the news about the locally-manufactured automatic centrifuge to the Imo State Health Management Board (HMB). I was subsequently invited by the Board for a demonstration of my P450 model. The Board Chairman, Dr Udemuo, and all the Board members were delighted to observe the efficiency of particulate sedimentations produced by the P450. The Board went into session and later called me in for a word. The chairman said, 'We have fully deliberated on your fantastic achievement. It was a pleasant surprise to many of us that a young Nigerian engineer from our own state could design and manufacture such a complicated medical device. The HMB has therefore decided to give you the encouragement you need at this crucial moment to build upon what you have already achieved'.

The HMB later authorised the purchase of two P450s for use in two of the Imo State outpost local government laboratories. The Board paid me the sum of ₦5000 for this transaction. The money realised from these initial sales was enough to enable me to modify the P450 and register a 'spin-off' company, Pokaiz Engineering Limited.

I really adored the two people who funded my university undergraduate and Master's Degree education, Chubuks and Papa; hence the company name, Hippolite-Chukwuebuka-Izume, or Pokaiz Engineering Limited. It later designed and manufactured other centrifuge models such as P300, P350, the P400 and a microhaematocrit centrifuge. These were marketed using the brand name 'Polite'.

My amiable Auntie Beatty was now speaking to a number of her laboratory scientist colleagues about the fantastic products her nephew was producing. I was to face the reality of marketing products which as yet had little reputation. I needed more powerful help in order to become visible and recognisable.

Auntie Beatty introduced me to her friend, Mr Emeka. Emeka was one of the most successful medical laboratory systems marketers in the state of Imo where I was settling. He was later to become a joint partner in my company, Pokaiz Engineering Limited. He was trained in the United States of America and had returned to Nigeria to set up his company, Chemitherm Nigeria Limited. At the time of partnering with Emeka, Chemitherm was already a household name amongst many medical laboratories across the entire southeast of Nigeria. Emeka admired my hard work and vision and supported me in no small measures for the spread of the application of 'polite' systems across the southeast of Nigeria.

Forming a company

I formally incorporated Pokaiz Engineering Limited in January 1994 after two years of operating under Emeka's company, Chemitherm Nigeria Limited. Emeka remained a co-director of the new production company. I was happy to allow Chemitherm Nigeria Limited to retain the marketing rights of the laboratory systems being designed and produced by Pokaiz Engineering Limited (PEL). By 1995, there were many systems in the range of laboratory products I was manufacturing at PEL, and they gradually gained a good reputation amongst Nigerian medical laboratory scientists and the systems were now in use in many cities in Nigeria, so I was invited to exhibit my products at the national conferences of the Nigeria Medical Laboratory Scientists.

Notable among these conferences was the 1995 one in the southern Nigerian city of Calabar. There were plenary session attestation remarks about the efficacy of the Polite systems by some senior Nigerian scientists who had used these products in their practices. The Association specifically asked two scientists who had previously used my services to present their remarks on the products. These were Dr Nanson from Abuja Specialist Hospital (northern Nigeria) and Mr Agwu from the Quality Control Laboratory of Groomy Gunner Breweries Umuahia (southern Nigeria). Both men had used a vast number of the machines in their departmental laboratories. Five units of three different models of the laboratory centrifuges were in use at the Abuja centre. The centre also had Polite laboratory incubators and waterbaths. The Quality Control Lab of the Umuahia brewery had used some of these products extensively as well.

Dr Nanson and Mr Agwu delivered very positive reports on the products, leading to much positive reaction from the attendees. It was a morale-boosting outing for me. Pokaiz Engineering Limited and I were becoming more popular and more confident in research, sourcing more avenues for the further development of the product range.

I refuse to compromise

During the early years, in association with Mr Emeka of Chemitherm Nigeria Limited, another notable marketer and exporter from the Eyimba-city of Aba, Conicon Nigeria Limited, also became interested in the products. Conicon exported reagents and laboratory devices to neighbouring West African countries such as Cameroon. The director of Conicon

Ltd approached us and negotiated for the right to export the Polite systems to other West African countries. Every part of the negotiation was easily agreed upon – except one. The systems were of a high quality and so perfectly finished that many doubted that they were really produced in Nigeria. This was during a time when made-in-Nigeria products hardly existed, or were castigated for their inferiority. For this reason the Conicon director did not want the 'made in Nigeria' label on his own items for export; instead he wanted them labelled 'made in China'. My colleagues did not see anything wrong with this request, since the products were indeed flawless and could easily be mistaken for those made in China, but they could not convince me that this was the right way to go. When I refused, Conicon threatened to pull out of the deal because they argued that Africa had no reputation for such products, and that Nigerian-branded products would be difficult to market. It was a big issue for me, as I argued that Nigeria needed to compete proudly in the open African market. The negotiation crumbled and Conicon withdrew their application, so I once again faced great frustration. It was an opportunity missed, but I never regretted my faith in African technological freedom.

After a couple of months another round of talks with Conicon resumed to explore a better way of managing the disagreement. It was finally agreed that my private conviction must be respected. Hence, the common ground solution was to label the systems as 'Manufactured for Nigeria by Pokaiz Engineering Limited'. Conicon hesitated but later accepted this. My products became export systems via Conicon Nigeria Limited, but the relationship lasted only four years.

Consultancy projects

The resulting successes brought more challenges as academic and scientific institutions began to ask me for technical assistance. Some awarded me contracts to devise improvised local-content modules as alternative spare parts to repair a large range of broken-down laboratory equipment for which spare parts were not available. The study of such systems – what they did and how they did it, as explained by the user scientists – soon gave me an insight into how I might devise methods of unravelling the failed components. The unavailability of spare parts for these failed assemblies eventually led to the development of a new skill, and the widening of my technical abilities. I would search for the best locally available components, whether sold separately or as an integral part of an easily affordable system in the local market, adapting these using interfaces to replace malfunctioning components in very expensive medical systems. The profit margins from such consultancies were often very lucrative, especially when this was done for big institutions, yet it was also a period of uncertainty, tension and hope as repaired systems were often given a technical warranty of up to six months of usage, and in a few cases up to 12 months.

The successes of this period brought more recognition, so bigger challenges emerged. The notable organisations and government agencies that my consultancies or laboratory systems served included the Eastern Nigeria regional headquarters of UNICEF, various departmental laboratories of the Federal University of Technology Owerri, the Quality Control Laboratory of the Groomy Gunner Breweries (GGB) Umuahia and the Water Laboratory of the Abia State Public

Utility Board, to mention only a few. I had now developed a huge amount of skill and had become very confident at searching local markets for components that I could easily re-engineer to replace a failed part of unrelated equipment. This skill was rare, so my fame quickly spread across the country, up to the Specialist Hospital Gwagwalada (SHG), Abuja FCT.

A remarkable early event that tested my skill and strength happened at the GGB Umuahia. Mr Hanz was a German expatriate and the Brewmaster at the company. The Quality Control Laboratory of the brewery had a malfunctioning piece of equipment used in the laboratory test-brewing of malt products. The system had been faulty even before Mr Hanz's arrival. The company was in dire need of test-running new samples and formulae from collaborating companies overseas to avoid the industrial scale wastage that could occur when products were presumptuously mass produced. There had been failed attempts to repair the system locally.

Mr Hanz and the Management of GGB considered the available options for the restoration of the laboratory device. It was a necessity that preproduction laboratory tests of intended malt products were carried out regularly as required by standards. It would cost a huge amount of money to fly in a German engineer to fix the malfunctioning laboratory brewer or replace the machine outright with a brand new imported system.

During one of the management meetings as the dilemma went on, Mr Eugene (Ezeugo), one of the senior management staff, turned to the Head of the Laboratory and said, 'We have this young engineer from the city of Owerri who has been fixing and servicing our centrifuges and autoclaves over the last eighteen months. Could he not be of any help to fix this system?'

Before Mr Agwu, the Head of the Laboratory, could say a word, the German brewmaster cut in, saying: 'Oh no, this is far more complicated than the centrifuge. I don't believe any Nigerian engineer could understand the complex engineering of the system, let alone fix the problem. Let's not waste our time looking for the solution where we will not find it'. Mr Hanz would not let anyone persuade him about this. After another round of deliberation, the Managing Director, Mr Ken, summarised the situation by saying: 'If there are no serious consequences in a trial, I will give approval for the engineer to be called to make an attempt; provided his estimated cost of repair is not too high. We can allow him some time and then move forward with any other options we can afford'.

Mr Hanz did not much like this idea, but he had no choice. He was however, confident that bringing in a Nigerian engineer would be a waste of time, saying the engineer would find no spare parts for this old equipment in this country and was bound to fail.

So I was invited to go ahead after a cost was agreed. It would be a couple of weeks before I could complete my work. Mr Hanz waited to be proved right. The laboratory scientist who was directly in charge of the system, Mr Johnson, spent a long time with me describing how the machine operated when it was in good working order. With my usual ingenious method of searching the local market, I picked up machine components that could provide the various actuations and outputs I needed to activate the aspects of the machine I believed were non-responsive. It was pleasant for the MD to hear that the cost of the entire repair was less than 8% of the cost of a brand new one or flying in a German engineer to fix the faulty machine. He gave his approval without hesitation for the repair contract to be awarded.

I chose to apply a very simple repair technique that would require some manual operation of a few process switches, just to keep cost down. Originally, these switches had operated automatically. The system worked very well during trial; however, the programming module of the system slightly distorted the sequencing of operation. Accordingly, the final product functioned slightly differently from what was expected. The laboratory scientist, Mr Johnson, was excited that the machine could deliver the expected product and would not mind the small distortion in sequencing. He later wrote a report stating his satisfaction with the repair.

When I submitted my claim for payment, it was processed but payment would not be made for another three weeks as Mr Hanz's certification was required for this. The excitement however ended when the Brewmaster returned and rejected the work. 'It must be 100% perfect before it can be accepted,' insisted Mr Hanz. He invited me for discussion and made it clear that the repair was unacceptable unless the device operated fully in 'automatic' mode. 'I predicted that you would not understand the sequencing but my colleagues would not listen to me,' said Mr Hanz.

'No, I fully understood about the sequencing distortion but I did not go into this because of the high cost of building a replacement semi-automatic module,' I said.

'And where will you get that from?' questioned Mr Hanz.

'I will create it,' I said confidently. 'I know the sequencing and timing, so I can construct a proper actuator interface to allow my new creation to take over the programming.'

Mr Agwu, the Deputy Brewmaster, who also served as the Head of Laboratory section, looked on in amazement as I faced his German boss. 'A new generation of Nigerian engineers has arisen and I am so proud of this,' Mr Agwu whispered to another colleague and smiled, looking at me. Turning towards the Brewmaster with a nod of approval, Mr Agwu chimed in: 'Hmm, this sounds hopeful'. But Mr Hanz would not give in.

I reported the sad encounter to Ezeugo, the Production Manager. Ezeugo was fast becoming a great motivator to me as he admired my ingenuity.

'Don't worry Hippolite, I will speak to the MD about this as I think you should be allowed to conclude with your ideas since you have already made some reasonable progress,' said Mr Ezeugo.

The long process of argument and Mr Hanz's arrogant attitude were highly demoralising, arousing my fighting spirit and determination to reject the devaluing of my ideas by Hanz. I had now made up my mind to inflate the cost of this extra job as a punishment for Mr Hanz's insults to my technical ability. I tried to explain to Mr Hanz the higher cost implications of restoring the system to a fully or semi-automated one.

'I have said it before and I say it again, you are not able to create this automation,' said Hanz. 'This is not the kind of engineering Nigerians can handle. I don't mind how much it costs. If you wish to do it, then payment can only come after I am satisfied with the sequencing and the delivered malt sample passes all the tests.'

My eyes were fixed on Mr Hanz as he gave his high-handed orders. 'Okay. I will do as you desire,' I said.

The decision was finally taken that I would produce a replacement module for the automation of the device as I claimed I could. There was such tension between the Brewmaster and me that I declared a state of 'no confidence' in any future assessment of the work by Mr Hanz. I argued that the German would not accept my work even if it was well done. It therefore became necessary for the MD to ask Mr Hanz to submit the details of his expected outputs from the device once properly repaired. Mr Hanz complied. The completed machine would be test-run before the company management team and all interested parties using three known products and sets of raw materials. The system would be operated by Mr Johnson in the presence of the Brewmaster and his Deputy.

I completed my work and a day was set for the testing. Everyone had a copy of the Brewmaster's list of expected outputs. The device was initially set on a dummy run for proof of automatic sequencing. This was completed satisfactorily, so they progressed to product brew-testing. At the end of all the semi-automated procedures involving three different formulae, the malt products were ready for testing. The results came out and all the boxes in the laboratory benchmark tables were ticked as within proper range; every aspect was satisfactory. Everyone was happily shaking my hand and saying, 'well done, I am proud of you; this is what Nigeria needs in this generation.'

As I had earlier resolved, I submitted a quotation that included a surcharge for the extra grilling and rough-handling by Mr Hanz. The extra profit margin would be handy for servicing my other pressing important needs; it was an exciting moment for me.

Mr Agwu was very proud of this outcome. Everything went as I demanded. The company paid me a huge sum of money.

After three years of running successful consultancy services at their various laboratories, Mr Agwu and Dr Nason, Head of the Department of Medical Laboratories at the Specialist Hospital Gwagwalada, were both happy to travel to the city of Calabar to present attestation remarks on the Polite laboratory systems at the national scientific conference of the Association of Medical Laboratory Scientists of Nigeria. Mr Agwu had been thrilled by the ingenuity I had displayed at GGB Umuahia in the preceding years.

The Nigerian Society of Engineers

My fame continued to soar, and the President of the Nigerian Society of Engineers (NSE), Dr Ehiman, was delighted to get to know me. Later in 1997 the Nigerian Society of Engineers invited Pokaiz Engineering Limited to the city of Abuja to display its range of laboratory systems at the first-ever Nigeria Technology Summit. This was attended by top government officials, captains of industry and educational and research institutions in Nigeria. It was an opportunity for many governmental figures and allied scientific professionals across Nigeria to admire my emerging talent through these products. Many of the individuals who visited PEL's stand made a number of notable remarks that became an added motivation to my entrepreneurial progress (see appendix 1). The Deputy President of the NSE, Chief Nanma, who would soon take over from Dr Ehiman, resolved to do everything necessary to encourage this emerging talent whenever he assumed office.

Chief Nanma would play a vital role in the later battles I had to fight to save Nigerian babies.

Humbled

More and more people were beginning to contact me to enquire about the scope of my consultancy services and my product range. A good number of medical laboratory departments from teaching hospitals in Nigeria had suffered from many years of inability to repair their broken-down equipment. Knowledge of my abilities was a relief, and some of them now began to invite me to inspect these systems. Lots of people respected and admired my talent and my emerging skills, which motivated me to do more.

There were, however, other prominent individuals who did the exact opposite, often making me wonder if I was wasting my time. Regarding my top class Bachelor's and Master's degrees in Mechanical Engineering, I had attractive credentials for the booming oil and gas industry in Nigeria. The snobbish attitude of some healthcare professionals tempted me to abandon my ambition to break new ground and use my degrees to get a decent job in the oil industry. The medical directors and chief medical directors at some of the hospitals I was invited to visit questioned if I had the right academic qualifications to practise within the medical field. Some were fond of creating strange scenes that seemed to suggest that I was inferior, as I had never taken a degree course in medicine at the university. I was naïve at times and was made to feel academically inferior during those early days. It was as if I did not have what it took to discuss the subject of medicine, let alone practise any aspect of it.

Then I was invited to see Dr Landus, the Medical Director of a tertiary hospital in the city of Ikom, southern Nigeria, to discuss the possibility of my helping to fix faulty laboratory systems at his tertiary hospital. I was immediately struck by his intimidating look. No sooner had I attempted to sit than Dr Landus stared at me as if the wrong person had come in and asked: 'Did they say you can fix our systems'?

'Yes sir, I can try,' I replied.

'Hmmm, where were you trained?' asked Dr Landus.

'I studied at Anambra State University of Technology Enugu,' I replied.

'Here in Nigeri-ya – and you say you can fix our systems? Listen, our systems are sophisticated machines that cost a huge amount of money to purchase. They are government property which must not be toyed with. The systems are not for every Tom, Dick and Harry to try their hands at fixing. These are machines for highly-trained professionals to handle – professionals trained in reputable countries and companies. Countries spend big money to educate those who do top jobs and sending them to top universities. For example, this country has spent a huge amount of money to train me in the United Kingdom and other countries for my various degrees in order to acquire the great skills I now possess as a top surgeon and as the Chief Medical Director of a teaching hospital. I mean top universities like Manchester, where I was trained. Have you heard of Manchester University – The great University of Manchester, England?'

'No sir,' I replied, intimidated and shaken.

'This is what you require to build your skills before you attempt to cause further damage to expensive medical equipment that you have never handled in the past. I am sorry but you can't do anything for us, young man.'

What is wrong with being trained in Nigeria? Must I acquire a foreign degree to be a good professional? These were the kinds of questions that resonated in my mind on the bumpy four-hour drive back to my home city of Owerri.

The neonatal crisis – face to face with neonates and MDG4

Some senior medical laboratory scientists paid attention to the skills I was displaying across the country and wanted more of their colleagues to have the opportunity of seeing me and my laboratory products in person. In March 1996, my company was invited to exhibit the systems in the southern city of Bayesa.

Unknown to me as I prepared to travel with my products to Bayesa for the 1996 annual scientific conference of the Association of Medical Laboratory Scientists of Nigeria (AMLSN), the Department of Paediatrics of nearby Mbong Teaching Hospital (MTH) was undergoing a period of remarkable change. The United Nations' Millennium Development Goal Target No. 4 on child survival (MDG4) had been launched in Nigeria and was gradually getting serious attention in the tertiary hospitals across the country. The mortality rate of children under five years of age (U5), including newly-born babies had to be reduced by 67% before 2015. Expectations were high for the paediatrics departments of hospitals across the nation to reduce the high neonatal mortality rates. Departmental leaders were faced with huge tasks and tests of their competence. Taking office as a Head of Department (HOD) of Paediatrics was no longer necessarily attractive, because of the fear of failure to achieve the set goals. This was a time that called for faculty men and women of boldness and personal confidence, whether divinely or arrogantly motivated.

The office of Head of Department at MTH became vacant, but who was to take over at such an undesirable period as this? Dr Kumara, a young, enthusiastic and passionate paediatrician who claimed a personal relationship with God, would accept the nomination provided his colleagues at the Department fasted and prayed for 21 days with him. This was his condition for acceptance of the office. So the faculty members gathered every evening to pray for the progress of the Department for the set 21 days. As they ended the long period of spiritual exercise, Kumara believed that God had given him an assurance that the most dreaded aspect of the job, which was neonatal survival, would turn out to be a success. This related to many years of total breakdown of all incubators at their Special Care Baby Unit (SCBU). Kumara had no clue whatsoever about how this would be achieved, having witnessed endless companies coming to MTH over the years to try to repair the incubators but being unable to fix any of the eight systems. The young consultant paediatrician assumed office as the new Acting Head of Department, but he was still confused as to how he could ever transform the neonatal outcomes of the SCBU without functional incubators.

Uncle Boba was an erudite senior engineer who lived in the city of Bayesa at the time. I had known uncle Boba for a couple of years. His great wisdom and love for younger professionals fostered a mentorship relationship from which I benefitted immensely. Boba was also a mentor to Dr Kumara at the time, although Kumara and I never knew each other.

A few days after Kumara assumed office as the new HOD, he visited Boba at his residence and told him of his initial spiritual exercise and how he had inner confidence of being successful with the incubators in the Special Care Baby Unit. Uncle Boba listened with keen interest, characteristically closing and opening his eyes as though he was silently communicating with another person in the spirit.

Dr Kumara continued: 'I am actually wondering how God would make this dream come true; I honestly do not know who it is that God would use to accomplish this for us, but...' Just then the telephone beside Boba began to ring and he picked it up. The caller was me.

'Hello uncle, this is Hippolite, I am calling from the city of Owerri,' I said.

'Ah brother Hippolite, please hold on a moment,' said uncle Boba. Turning to Kumara and using the palm of his hand to cover the telephone mouthpiece, he said, 'I think I know whom the Lord would use to deliver the success you talked about – he is the one on the phone now. God is never late, is He?' He then turned around to continue with the telephone call.

Dr Kumara remained ecstatic with excitement, eagerly waiting for Uncle Boba to finish the call. I explained to Boba how I had planned to come to Bayesa the very next week to honour an invitation as an exhibitor at the AMLSN annual scientific conference. I promised to visit the senior engineer during the trip. Uncle Boba however re-emphasised to me that it was a good thing I was coming to Bayesa because there was another crucial challenge I might have to tackle, for Mbong Teaching Hospital in the neighbouring city.

Dr Kumara and I were later introduced to each other at the home of Uncle Boba, and this marked the beginning of a professional friendship between the two enthusiastic and ambitious young professionals, Kumara and me.

CHAPTER 3

A VISION TAKES SHAPE

✦✦✦✦✦✦✦

Iknew little about Millennium Development Goal number 4 (MDG4) and how this related to Kumara's new job at the time. Dr Kumara educated me on the challenges and expectations, explaining how it was not possible to achieve any success without functional incubators, as was the situation at MTH Mbong. He conducted me round his Special Care Baby Unit (SCBU) facility, showing me the eight faulty incubators and the hapless new-born babies being managed with the use of 'hardware hot water bottles' to keep them warm in the cots and broken-down incubators.

'This is an ineffective and crude method of maintaining the

body temperature of a newborn baby, but we have no choice,' Dr Kumara said sadly.

'How long has this been going on?' I asked.

'As long as I can remember. I cannot remember a time when we had all our incubators working. For over ten years, countless companies have tried to fix them without success. The hospital has managed to purchase one or two new ones, but these soon failed and joined the piles of malfunctioning lots you see right here in the Unit and the others you are yet to see at the store of the Maintenance Workshop.'

I was moved with compassion when Kumara added: 'For this reason, many of our extremely premature babies do not make it, sadly'.

'Do you mean they die?' I asked.

'Yes, it is very rare for any neonate below 1000g at birth to survive without a functioning incubator; most or all of them will die,' Kumara replied.

I was suddenly moved by extreme feelings of compassion and sadness. I began to wonder what could make it so hard to fix these neonatal incubators for these poor babies.

'Any reason for the failure of these companies you said had come to try to fix the incubators?' I asked.

'The excuse was often given as lack of spare parts, but they still achieved no success even when this was not the case. We think the incubator is too complicated for our Nigerian engineers to handle,' said Kumara.

Thoughts about the technology behind the functioning of neonatal incubators began to occupy my mind. I thought they might not be too different from that of laboratory incubators and hot air ovens. I was already producing these and laboratory waterbaths in my product range at Pokaiz Engineering, although I had no idea of the unique characteristics of the neonatal incubator.

'I do not want to disappoint you, but I have never handled this kind of system,' I said. 'If you don't mind, I will spend some time studying neonatal incubators, and then carefully examine the control unit of one of these before attempting any restoration. This will take weeks though.'

Kumara was happy with this suggestion, so I detached the control unit from an Airshields Isolette model C86 incubator and left for Owerri.

Owerri, the capital city of Imo State, was predominantly occupied by the highly enterprising Igbo tribe, popularly known as 'Ndi Igbo'. The central library was rich in scientific books, including life sciences. I was able to obtain books that enabled me to understand the basic capabilities and features of a functional neonatal incubator. I also privately studied the constituent assemblies of the incubator and how these interacted with each other to deliver their functions. My technical knowledge of the laboratory incubator was an added advantage, as this enabled me to gain a fairly quick understanding of how the infant incubator worked.

After two weeks of studying, it was time to open up the power pack unit I had brought back from MTH Mbong. I studied the various components and circuitry of the Narco-Airshields Isolette system. Based on the theories from the books I had studied, I was able to identify the components that seemed to be failing to deliver their functions. I had to find replacements for these, but where?

During similar dilemmas in the past, the Igbo city of Aba (also known as Enyimba City) had proved handy for sourcing components. The great entrepreneurial skills of the Igbo people were showcased in their numerous commercial businesses across the entire Nigerian nation. With these they had built the largest West African market city of Onitsha and also the commercial city of Aba, popularly known for the manufacture of many made-in-Nigeria goods. A lot of cottage metal fabrication workshops were dotted across the south-eastern Igbo cities of Aba, Enugu and Awka. There were also marketers of industrial elements, machine controls and components of all kinds in these cities. Some traders specialised in marketing brand new components for common machine systems, while others traded in components recycled from old machines. These were sold in designated areas of the town referred to as 'akpakara-dimgbom,' an Igbo phrase for 'scrap components'. This rich aspect of the Igboland was a great support for what I would later do for the Nigerian neonates. I combed the cities of the Igboland, searching from shop to shop and from one akpakara-dimgbom marketer to another. I was looking for the best equivalents of all the components I wished to replace in the MTH incubator system I was working on.

Alterations were made, and finally the power-pack unit responded as I expected. This was an exciting time in my life. It had taken weeks of sleepless nights and hard work, motivated by one passion – to end the misery of the deaths suffered by the tiny newborns I had seen at Mbong.

Had all the hard work paid off? This was yet to be determined, by another trip to the small city of Mbong. This time the aim was to install the powerpack back in its main incubator, and to commence technical and perhaps clinical tests to confirm its functionality.

I picked up the telephone and dialled Dr Kumara's number. 'I have good news for you,' I said. 'The powerpack is now running the way I expected it to run.'

'Oh that's fantastic! So we should be expecting you at Mbong very soon?' Kumara enquired.

'Sure, in fact I'm coming in the next two days as I am as curious as you are in this matter. I'm excited, but I don't want to celebrate until I confirm that the new interfaces will fit into the main incubator and generate the expected outputs.'

The rigorous technical and clinical testing lasted three days. Kumara and his colleagues were finally satisfied that the Isolette C86 system was running and delivering as expected, and it was now time to celebrate. Kumara assembled his management team and invited the chief medical director, Dr Kamilus, to his official unveiling of the 're-programmed' incubator. This was a huge achievement for the young consultant, who had assumed office as the Acting HOD only a couple of months earlier. Dr Kumara's fame spread across the whole MTH, with messages of congratulation for bringing back hope for the Special Care Baby Unit. The hardworking Kumara was able to persuade the MTH management to provide funding for gradual but steady re-programming of the rest of the broken-down incubators using the same technique, until they were all restored. The six months of warranty and free back-up support for the operation of the systems were successful and free of serious technical hitches.

Kumara also encouraged his hospital to enter into a long consultancy relationship via a formal maintenance agreement mutually signed by MTH and Pokaiz Engineering Limited. Thus, MTH became the first Nigerian tertiary hospital to sign a formal SCBU agreement with Pokaiz Engineering Limited, appointing me as a visiting technical consultant to the Unit.

'You will soon understand that MTH is not alone in this ugly problem, as every single tertiary hospital in this country is faced with this same problem; I guess you will be happy to help other hospitals too,' Kumara said as he escorted me to my car during one of the early visits following my new appointment.

'I wish I could save all the neonates with my small knowledge of incubator systems,' I replied.

My friendship with Kumara lasted many years, even after Kumara left office as the Head of the Department of Paediatrics. His successful tenure aided his rapid promotion and professional progress; I contributed in no small measure to this. Kumara later served as the MTH Chairman of the Medical Board, which made him the second in command in the management team of the entire hospital. He was later appointed Professor of Paediatrics and Chief Medical Director of another tertiary hospital, the Otungo Teaching Hospital (OTH) in Benue State. Kumara's success rubbed off on my progress, because Kumara's professional colleagues from other tertiary hospitals heard of the successes and wanted to know more about Pokaiz Engineering Limited and the man behind the incubator re-programming technique.

The first 24 months of dedicated technical support and preventive maintenance of the incubators at MTH Mbong was an invaluable period of learning for me. My confidence and practical understanding of the neonatal incubator was enhanced as I observed the doctors and nurses at work. Soon I was able to understand how to translate a desirable thermal condition for a neonate into a machine input function. I understood the importance of effective thermal calibration of the incubator, without which the babies could not be well supported.

This period of learning also revealed that the inadequate understanding of the operation of a fully functional incubator by clinicians and nurses was an adverse factor affecting neonatal survival. I now had to find a way of teaching the doctors and nurses. I wanted to know the specific neonatal and machine parameters that interacted, and the definition of any transfer-function required to determine how a specific machine input would produce a desired neonatal output.

My questions sounded too complex for the doctors, so they yielded no immediate answers. I would have to study to develop the right answers to these questions. The training curriculum of Nigerian doctors and nurses emphasised the importance of adequate neonatal thermoneutral control; however, there were no teaching modules dedicated to how this could be effectively achieved with an incubator. Hence, manipulation of the incubator or the 'hardware hot water bottle' for the thermal stability of the neonate had no standard algorithm and was left at the discretion or the limit of understanding of the attendant on duty. This exposed the neonates as perpetual 'guinea pigs', as every attendant manipulated the incubator by trial and error techniques. Suffice to say that a lot of tiny babies lost their lives to this knowledge-gap. Why was such a vital aspect of intervention for keeping babies alive so ignored during the training of nurses and doctors? Why had no one found a way of stopping this trial and error approach? Could this be one of the reasons why so many Nigerian neonates died? These questions occupied my mind all the time.

Challenge at Asaba – PIT course established

Doctor Kumara spoke to his colleagues at other leading teaching hospitals, notably Eastern City Teaching Hospital (ECTH) Asaba, which led to more invitations and successful outings. At ECTH I met the Head of Department, Professor Norman, a professor of neonatology, who would later become a long friend and mentor, motivating me as I advanced my knowledge in medical engineering and development of devices for neonatal care. There were six broken-down incubators that no company or the in-house maintenance department were able to fix at Professor Norman's hospital. The ugly story was similar to MTH's, as Kumara had rightly hinted.

Professor Norman introduced me to his SCBU Head of Unit, Dr Gabus. Gabus was a man with a big chest and large frame who had previously served in the military. He and his other colleagues at the SCBU had been told that the engineer behind the success at MTH Mbong would be coming to examine their systems. The demand for military precision and discipline in the army had truly rubbed off on Dr Gabus and his desire to succeed in medical practice. In their previous trials for possible repair options, the maintenance department would invite any person who claimed to be able to fix the incubators. Many of these would remove the system from the hospital and keep it in their workshops for a long time without repairing it successfully, often returning the system with missing parts. Gabus and his colleagues had seen many failed attempts like this, so they took the new promises from the young engineer from the city of Owerri with a pinch of salt. Gabus narrated how they had ensured that every incubator that had been removed for repairs was brought back in anticipation of my visit.

As he drove to work one day, Dr Gabus spotted someone wheeling an incubator towards the ECTH main gate. Gabus had already driven into the compound and was close by, so he quickly found a parking slot, jumped out of the car and raised his right hand high. In a booming military voice, he yelled: 'Hey man, stop there!'

As he approached the man with the incubator he raised his voice again: 'who are you and where are you taking that machine?'

'Engineer Anyaukwu of the maintenance department has authorized me to take this machine to my workshop in town to attempt its repairs,' the man replied.

'All right, I am the consultant in charge of that SCBU,' bellowed Dr Gabus. 'Before I close my eyes and open them again, you had better return this system back to the Unit.'

The intimidating look in Gabus's eyes was so frightening that the man did not even let him finish the command before he turned back to return the incubator.

It took two weeks for me to complete the re-programming of all the six incubators. I also carried out my schedules for functionality tests and was happy with the performance of the systems, and they all demonstrated to Professor Norman and his departmental team. I engaged Dr Gabus in discussions during the course of the re-programming exercise to understand how much practical experience of the use of functional incubators existed with the current team of doctors and nurses at the SCBU.

'I must be very honest with you that I do not have a good level of knowledge,' said Dr Gabus. 'I know that none of my colleagues might be any better. These systems never worked for the many years we have been in this Unit. Any theoretical and practical knowledge of this device will go a long way for us. You may have to incorporate staff training as you prepare your bills for the hospital, but you need to speak to the Chief Medical Director about this first.'

The MTH Mbong experience showed me that staff training in paediatric incubation techniques would have to become a key factor as attendants changed from the use of 'hot water bottles' to proper functioning incubators. I was not an academically certified doctor, so I was not really qualified to teach a clinically-biased audience, but there was no other person as knowledgeable as me to develop and teach this course. I had already been developing such a course module after I had learned the knowledge level of the clinicians and nurses at MTH Mbong. Professor Norman and his entire department were happy for this training course to be completed before the commissioning of the re-programmed incubators. However, Dr Akabon, the CMD, felt otherwise.

I had been ushered into his large office to hold a discussion on the need for the paediatrics incubation techniques course. Dr Akabon was instantly furious with me when I said that the doctors and nurses needed to undergo some training before the commissioning of the restored incubators. The CMD looked up, removed his reading glasses and stared at me. 'And who would be the trainer?' he snapped.

As Akabon listened to me, the unknown non-medical person, talking about being a teacher to his consultants, he was full of rage and contempt: 'Who do you think you are and what qualifications do you possess to teach my doctors?' he asked. It was obvious that many years of seeing engineers who had tried and failed to solve this problem had led Akabon to expect no chance of success from me, even after the news that the restored incubators had passed their functionality tests. Why was Dr Akabon looking down on me like this way, or did he think the repaired systems would not last?

At last, the CMD turned to me. 'Young man, I have finished with you, as I will not accept your proposal,' he said. 'You have not got what it takes to train my doctors. How dare you presume to be so skilled?'

Now boiling inside, I replied: 'Okay then, I need to warn you that you do not have my permission to use those incubators, because your doctors and nurses could kill babies with them instead of saving them. You may send for me when you are ready'.

I reported this sad encounter to Professor Norman, the Head of the Paediatrics Department, and departed for Owerri. As I journeyed home, the questions in my mind were endless. I kept wondering why doctors did not seem to respect the fact that I too was a graduate, with six years of post-MSc qualification in Engineering. Did I have to have a medical degree to be an effective teacher for a doctor who did not know how to handle these medical systems for adequate support to these dying babies? Why didn't it seem to bother some people that these tiny babies were dying? Could such administrative bullying be one of the reasons why so many Nigerian neonates had died?

The Paediatrics Department later filed an official demand to the Management of ECTH stating that they would not put the machines to use unless the training took place. This departmental pressure finally led to another meeting, when Dr Akabon was reconciled with me and the training was arranged.

The three days of training was a huge success. All participants testified that the training was of very high quality – far beyond what they expected. One of the trainees who had just passed his final residency exams from the SCBU, Dr Buisi, gave a vote of thanks, saying: 'I have been the chief resident doctor of the SCBU for all these years without any functional incubators. To me, an incubator had become a mystery box with unknown components, a system that made good technicians look foolish. When engineer Hippolite arrived to begin his incubator re-programming in our unit, dragging out and dismantling each system down to its components, without taking the systems to some magic workshop in town as we were used to, my colleagues and I mocked him. But when I saw the incubators working one after another, I changed my mind about this engineer; he must be a genius and a magician. After seeing the incubators work, I was determined not to miss the training even though the hospital couldn't fund every participant. I am glad I sourced private funding to attend this invaluable training and I am happy it happened within my last few weeks before final disengagement from this teaching hospital. Using such a simplified technique and with a master-class of teaching skill, our trainer has removed the aura and stigma that often made me see the incubator as a mystery box that must never be touched.'

The closing ceremony and award of certificates was attended by senior figures at the hospital, including a lady described as the icon of West African Paediatrics practice, Dr Kate, who was the director of the Institute of Child Health and a professional of high standing amongst her peers. In her remarks as the chairperson of the occasion she announced: 'Today I have had one of the biggest surprises of my professional career'. As the audience reacted to this declaration in amazement, she continued with a gesture: 'Oh Yeees!' – that a Nigerian engineer has been able to do the work which we always used to reserve for the foreign experts. Quite frankly, I never really believed that anybody in Nigeria would be able to come and repair our incubators, so Mr Hippolite, you are a new breed and a rare breed.'

Many of the cohorts of this inaugural 'Paediatric Incubation Techniques' course moved on to become highly successful in their various practices around Nigeria. Some went on to become my personal friends and met up again much later in their careers, some as directors of their tertiary hospitals or heads of the Department of Paediatrics.

I retained maintenance rights for the systems at ECTH for the entire duration of the 12 months of warranty. As the period was approaching an end, one of the senior nurses described her experience in a chat with me: 'This has by far been the sweetest period of my nursing career in this hospital, having fully functional incubators, and I hope they don't allow you to disappear at the end of it'.

I went to Professor Norman to announce my official disengagement at the end of the 12 months.

'Thank you Hippolite, it has been a great joy and an unforgettable pleasure having you on board,' said the Professor. 'Our department has officially applied to the hospital management to re-engage you as a 'visiting consultant' on a longer-term maintenance-agreement with your company.'

During the negotiations for the consultancy agreement, Dr Akabon expressed his happiness, explaining how he had almost missed the opportunity of having me to resolve the problem he had always had as the CMD. 'To me it was a done deal that you were going to be formally re-engaged as a visiting consultant to our hospital, but I still had one mystery to resolve,' he said. Everyone laughed and waited for his next words. Fixing his eyes on me, the CMD continued: 'I got more confused with you initially because I had heard you were an arrogant man.' Dr Akabon stared at me while Professor Norman and others looked on. 'But in the last year I have carefully monitored your activities and relationships in this hospital. I have also waited for complaints from some of my staff who might notice your arrogance to confirm my previous impression, to no avail. Frankly, I don't seem to have seen any basis for this impression about your character, so I am really sorry for that initial misunderstanding between us'.

'No worries, sir, I understand,' I replied. 'However, there is only one man in the Nigerian healthcare system who could call me arrogant – I mean someone you could have easily met during your Nigerian CMD club meeting, who would want to defame my character.'

Professor Norman looked at me in bewilderment as Akabon, now smiling, asked: 'And who do you think this fellow could be?'

I hesitated, looking at my great friend Norman and then back at Akabon.

'Professor Nahosuwa of course, as I can't think of any other person in the entire country who could be doing this to defame me'.

Akabon looked away and said nothing.

Negotiations went well and deals were agreed upon; Dr Akabon did not hesitate to sign. Thus, ECTH Asaba became the second Nigerian tertiary hospital to sign an agreement with me after MTH Mbong.

In a later private discussion, Norman wanted to know more about the CMD's confusion about 'arrogance'. I narrated my ugly encounter with Professor Nahosuwa – a fight in the defence of my personal principles and the rights of the neonates. Nahosuwa was the Chief Medical Director of another tertiary hospital and he wanted to exploit my talents for his personal gain, offering to overspend government money through my work. He had not got his wish and so took to defaming me in order to discourage CMD club colleagues who might wish to offer me a job. The encounter with Professor Nahosuwa is fully described elsewhere in this book.

Neonatal survival at ECTH Asaba was now improving. The doctors, nurses and mothers were happy, but one section of the hospital was discontented – the Maintenance Department. The head of the Maintenance Section, Engr. Anyaukwu, and his team members at the section loved it when the systems were faulty and remained broken down. They regularly demanded money from the management to purchase components and parts which would do nothing to solve the problems of the crippled SCBU. They were so corrupt that they filled their pockets with cash, to the detriment of the poor dying babies. They never cared about the consequences of their actions, enjoying being addressed with the title of 'Engr' but having minds which were empty of technical expertise and full of nothing but corruption. My ingenuity had ended the years of misery they had imposed on the neonates, as well as the flow of ill-gotten money.

At the demand of the Paediatrics Department and the Head of Unit of the SCBU, the technicians were banned from touching the incubators all through the remaining years of Akabon's directorship. My ingenuity made a mockery of their intelligence and made them look greatly inferior in practice. In the usual manner, the doctors looked down on them. Anyaukwu and his men saw me as a threat that must be removed. They had to fight back, but they had to wait for the best opportunity.

Led by Anyaukwu, they waged a war of frustration on Pokaiz Engineering Limited (PEL) as soon as Akabon left office. The Nigeria federal government had just launched their operation 'due process,' which was being used in fighting corruption in the civil service. The so-called 'administrative due process' of the Nigerian government at the time became a good reason for Anyaukwu's unit to assume the responsibility of endorsing PEL's job certification before payment. This certification endorsement had all along been the duty of the user department (via the Head of the SCBU and the Head of Paediatrics Department). The new CMD felt that the 'Due Process' agenda would also require the Maintenance Section of the hospital to supervise and confirm that PEL had done their job satisfactorily.

The new CMD refused to pay attention to the experiences of his predecessor, Dr (now Professor) Akabon, and this was the opportunity the corrupt Anyaukwu and the maintenance technicians had been waiting for. They began to demand bribes before they would endorse PEL bills and certificates of job completion. This move frustrated and infuriated me, leading to several threats to withdraw my consultancy at the teaching hospital. The so-called maintenance men obviously loved money more than the survival of the neonates; one does not need to go too far to find the true enemies of those little babies. These greedy 'caterpillars' were the real reason why so many Nigeria neonates died.

CHAPTER 4

TACKLING THE NEONATES' ENEMIES

✦✦✦✦✦✦✦

Professor Norman was delighted to be the person who had brought me to ECTH in 1997, so he was instrumental to the hospital's success with me. He was prepared to use his influence as a top professional in Nigerian paediatric practice to make me known further afield. He used every opportunity during meetings to declare to colleagues: 'Based on our experience at ECTH, any SCBU that wanted to make an MDG(4) impact for neonates should send for this young engineer Hippolite'.

This led to more invitations from tertiary hospitals across the country and I had to find a way of accommodating these demands. Dr Kumara of MTH Mbong helped to secure an exhibition stand for PEL to display their laboratory product range during the 1997 annual scientific conference of the Paediatrics Association of Nigeria (PANConf) in the city of Otukpo. Kumara travelled together with me and my team and was a great support as he brought his professional colleagues to PEL's stand for introduction.

Invitations came from a number of tertiary hospitals after the successful PANConf 1997 outing. I tried to honour as many as I could. I was soon to discover how universally awful and corrupt the Nigerian healthcare system was. My passion to save the neonates and change the outcomes of SCBU often drove me to the point of extreme danger. I looked forward to discovering the technical reasons why the incubators failed, but ended up discovering further man-made reasons why Nigerian neonates died. I had come to realise how huge the problem of lack of functional incubators was. I wondered how this had become such an intimidating monster to a nation as large as Nigeria. I also realised that the incubator application was only one aspect of a whole lot of interventions needed for effective neonatal care. It did not take long before I understood that there were parallel challenges with other applications, such as respiratory distress syndrome (RDS), jaundice, sepsis, and so on. Applications and devices for these interventions had remained like magic boxes that only 'white witches' could handle.

The pressure began to mount from other clinicians, who felt that I could also devote my energies to these other applications. I felt an enormous sense of sympathy as I observed the struggles of respiratory-distressed babies. I wished I could look into this as well, but I had to concentrate on my incubator study in order to develop and properly validate a local-content solution for this.

The repeated breakdown of mechanical ventilators or outright lack of these applications to help distressed neonates were issues that kept being presented to me. Without mincing my words, I replied to one of the worried consultants: 'I fully understand the frustration. I have carefully observed that paediatricians are actually more worried about incubators than about these other equally important applications. If I do not concentrate on delivering a decisive solution on the incubators, I might end up achieving nothing. Respiratory distress would be my next stop after thermal distress.'

I needed to be firm and resolute in order to tackle the restoration of proper incubator care across the whole of Nigeria with my 'reprogramming' technique. The more invitations I received from centres across Nigeria, the more I was exposed to unacceptable practices and inappropriate behaviours, more reasons why Nigeria neonates were dying. I was determined to fight on for these babies.

Professor Ayubak, the CMD of the Savana Tertiary Hospital (STH) Wukari, who had trained under great Professor Norman of ECTH, heard of the Asaba success. He knew as a former resident doctor how bad the ECTH SCBU used to be, so he did not hesitate to ask me to come to the far northwest of Nigeria to help. All the incubators at the hospital were faulty except two newly-installed ones. This was quite inadequate to manage a large unit of up to 30 inmates with only two functional incubators. The hospital was still under pressure to get the failed systems working.

STH Wukari had a maintenance unit that was headed by an engineer called Mr Oke, who was such a greedy fellow that he reminded me of the dreaded character of Mr Anyaukwu at Asaba. He pretended to be happy that the hospital had finally found a knowledgeable engineer to tackle the incessant breakdown of incubators at the SCBU.

In order to follow government so-called 'due process,' Prof Ayubak asked Mr Oke to liaise closely with me so as to make my work at Savana hospital free of hitches. Professor Ayubak treated me so nicely, always acknowledging how well his former teacher, Professor Norman, had spoken about me. Mr Oke remained a good friend – until it was time for the hospital to pay for my services. Then he began to make comments and display body language that reminded me of the antics of Mr Anyaukwu of Asaba.

I was not prepared to get into this ugly business where technicians inflated the cost of jobs to enable them to steal money from the institution. I pretended not to understand Mr Oke's dirty game. I ignored Oke's advances until Oke decided to boldly ask me what cut of the cost of my services would be given to him.

'I don't understand. Are you asking me for a bribe before you process my papers for payment?' I asked.

'I am going to process the paper, of course,' said Oke. 'I am only making sure that I will be appreciated after you have received your payment; this is what every contractor does.'

Inappropriate behaviour of maintenance technicians like Mr Oke would normally compel contractors to offer some bribe in order to process the job-completion documents they needed to get payment. Contractors who refused to play ball were usually punished with payment delays or outright 'hiding away' of their contract files until a higher authority demanded them. Some very senior staff could often have a hand in this corrupt practice, and would turn a blind eye to the behaviour of the junior officers. Some of them would advise contractors to go and settle their issues with the juniors. I was happy that I could easily seek an audience with the CMD if the situation became unmanageable.

Mr Oke was greatly frustrating me, and doing everything he could to make money out of my consultancy. It would often take the intervention of Professor Ayubak to challenge Oke's excesses and get my bills paid to keep my consultancy alive. The greed of heads of maintenance units and their antagonism towards me for refusing to bribe them – the 'what's-in-it-for-me' syndrome – became a nightmare that resurfaced at every tertiary hospital where the incubator re-programming project was executed. I began to think of these people as greedy 'caterpillars' who could not stop feeding on the funds which were supposed to be used to save the neonates. As soon as these fellows realised that I was not prepared to pay them 'comrades-in-crime' money, they would challenge my ability to fix the systems. I really never bothered to butter up these money-loving, neonate-hating people. They were never humble enough to learn and would always try to pose as though they knew it all. 'If you really know this, why have you been unable to get these incubators working so as to save the countless dying babies?' I would usually ask them. Based on earlier experiences, I never allowed these 'maintenance gangs' any chance to intimidate me. I would always declare to them: 'I have got only one business in this hospital – and that is to save the neonates'. Sometimes I added: 'I am very happy to disappoint any other agenda you may present – whether by words, body languages or implied comments'.

Another disaster, another challenge

Maryland Training Hospital Akure was one of the most cherished Nigerian Federal Government-owned hospitals. In April 2000 a crisis erupted in its Special Care Baby Unit because a neonate died as a result of an incubator disaster. This exposed the appalling lack of functional incubators at the centre to the press. The news was everywhere, causing great embarrassment to the Federal Government of Nigeria. Both the chairman of the hospital management board, Professor Iboji, and the CMD, Professor Oluti, were under pressure to find anyone who could assist in fixing the problem. They knew the situation posed a threat to their jobs.

I travelled to Akure at the invitation of the chairman of the hospital, who had heard about my great successes and asked me to assess the incubators in the SCBU. The Chairman and CMD gladly welcomed me. I was later introduced to Mr Nika, the young maintenance engineer in-charge of the incubators. Nika was detailed to join me as I assessed the systems. In my usual compassion for the terrible suffering of the babies due to the broken-down equipment, I was groaning within and would not entertain any distracting discussions that were not connected to the incubators. This made Nika feel that his job, skills and intelligence were being challenged. He attempted various stunts to get me to become some kind of a friend in order to discuss the 'what's-in-it-for-me' aspect with him. I intentionally blocked every move to initiate such discussions, and tension began to run high. Nika's anxiety was becoming noticeable, and he started behaving as though I was an enemy who must be stopped. Nika was about my age and was always posing as a serious religious man, some kind of Christian. He always had a pocket-sized edition of the Holy Bible prominently stuck in his back pocket. One would have expected him to be different if he was truly a genuine Christian.

I was severely disappointed that even people of my own age were participating in the foolish game of dishonesty. I felt that I had fought older monsters for the neonates, and Nika was just small fry by comparison.

The assessments were concluded in quick time. I drafted my proposals and cost implications and submitted these to the CMD. The hospital management were pleased with the submission and a Job Order document was signed for PEL to repair two incubators using the re-programming technique at an agreed fee. The job was completed and the bill was submitted without delay for the payment to be processed. I ensured that all required documentation was submitted along with the bill and request-for-payment application.

Normally, payment cheques would be ready for collection within seven working days of submission of all relevant documents. However, there was a delay. Each time I enquired whether my cheque was ready for collection, the Accounts Department responded that no payment documents for Pokaiz Engineering Limited had been received, let alone processed.

I began to suspect that Nika had refused to prepare the job completion certification that was mandatorily required for payment to be processed. His immediate line manager, the

Director of Works, must have referred my documentations to him for his comments as a matter of 'due process' before the job completion certificate could be produced.

It was soon two months since I had completed the job and the incubators had been in full operation at the SCBU, but there was no sign of my payment. No one seemed to want to help me to navigate the difficult personnel at the hospital, because everyone seemed to seek financial gratification first. I could take this no more, so I decided to go to the clerical officers at the CMD's office.

'Is it possible to know what has happened to my application for payment which I submitted to the CMD nearly two months ago, please?' I asked one of the staff on duty.

'Have a seat,' said the officer, pointing to the chair opposite his desk. 'So, what is the name of your company?' He reached for the file movement register and began to search. With his finger pointed at a line in the register, he looked up to me and said: 'Okay, I can confirm that Pokaiz Engineering Limited papers have since been treated by the CMD and sent to the Works Department for verification and certification of job. This was dispatched to the Director of Works two days after it was submitted to the CMD. This paper must normally be returned to the CMD for him to authorise payment processing before it could be sent to the Accounts Department'.

Off I went to the Works Department. The clerical staff checked through the register and said the paper had been processed by the Director of Works, so it was no longer in their office. They could not trace exactly where the papers had been dispatched to. I suspected that they might have been sent to Nika. I knew this had all been orchestrated by Nika to put me under pressure to offer a bribe; it was a pattern I had seen over and over again.

Then Nika demanded that I should see him in his office for discussion. I flatly refused, saying, 'I do not engage with maintenance people on discussions outside neonatal technical issues. You saw me test and commission the systems and I can answer any other technical question you may have over the phone or at the SCBU in the presence of the doctors and nurses'.

'Okay then, if you feel too big to come and see me I will wait until you are ready,' said Nika.

'You have been sitting on my papers for too long,' I replied. 'I need to warn you that people don't toy with me. You need to be careful with me because God fights fiercely on my side – bible or no bible in your back pocket.'

Nika became angry. 'All right, we shall see,' he said.

I waited another three weeks, and still I was not paid. There was no point begging these immoral fellows; the only thing that could move them was an executive order from above, but how could that be arranged? Meanwhile the doctors and nurses at the SCBU were full of praise for the incubators, which had now been running satisfactorily for over three months. They discussed this in their meetings and demanded that the management should consider bringing back the young engineer to re-programme more of the malfunctioning incubators for them, as a good number of these were packed at one end of the SCBU. The Chairman of the Board of Management, who himself was a professor of paediatrics, was delighted with the success and reports coming from the Paediatrics department. He did not hide his admiration for me, and quickly asked for me to see him in his office. I was delighted with the Chairman's positive reactions.

'I am glad, sir, that the management and all the clinicians are appreciative of my hard work; however, I don't understand why the hospital has refused to pay me,' I said to the chairman.

'You don't mean that, do you?' said Professor Iboji, staring at me. 'You haven't been paid for the job yet?' he raised his voice.

'No sir, I was told that my file was missing so my papers have not been processed for payment up till this very moment,' I replied.

Professor Iboji was a man with a huge frame and an intimidating look. Turning away from me, he reached for the telephone and switched on its hands-free mode so his conversation could be heard by another person. He dialled the CMD.

'Hello sir,' answered the CMD.

'Oluti Oluti, why hasn't the young man Hippolite been paid for the good job he did for us three months ago?' Professor Iboji demanded with a harsh tone in his voice.

'Sir, I am told he has travelled, so...'

Before the CMD could stammer the next word, Professor Iboji said: 'He is still in the country and in fact, he has just called me and I asked him to come straight away and pick up his cheque. He is on his way to you right now, so make sure his cheque is ready for collection as soon as he arrives'.

The Chairman turned off the phone and said to me, 'Go right away to the CMD's office'.

As I was entering Professor Oluti's office, I saw the head of the Works Department, Mr Alani, rushing out of it towards his own office. The CMD saw me and asked me to exercise a little more patience. The CMD had quickly looked into what had happened and discovered that he had sent the papers to the Head of Works over two months earlier, so he had sent for Mr Alani and warned him of the possibility of a query on this issue. Mr Alani traced the file to Mr Nika, who was not at work on that day, so for fear of being queried by the CMD, Mr Alani instructed his staff to break open Nika's office to get the paper out. This was done and Mr Alani, without any hesitation, issued a query to Mr Nika, then quickly certified the work himself and took the file by hand straight to the CMD. Mr Alani also indicated to the CMD that Mr Nika had been asked to explain the delay. Within the next two hours, every protocol was hastily completed and I was asked to sign and collect my cheque.

A few days later, I called Nika and said: 'I hope by now you must know the answer to your query. In the future never toy with me or anyone who has God on his side, bible in your pocket or not'.

I was glad and grateful to God for this help. Yet although I was happy to have been paid, I remained sad as I wondered why some technicians were so unhelpful, why they were so boastful despite having little education and knowledge and why they preferred making money to saving neonates. Why did it take such an executive force to get a simple thing done for these poor innocent neonates? The questions in my mind were endless.

I next set off to the ancient city of Isoko. I had gone to honour an invitation from the Midwest Tertiary Hospital (MWTH), which had piles of broken-down incubators that could not be repaired by the in-house maintenance staff. Such a situation was no longer any surprise to me – all referral hospitals in Nigeria, no doubt, were suffering the same problem. I had become used to visiting a centre to be shown several malfunctioning incubators being used as bed spaces for neonates, or stuffed with hot water bottles to provide warmth. It would have been a pleasant surprise for me to be shown a fleet of functional incubators anywhere in Nigeria, so I was always prepared for the worst case each time I visited a hospital.

At the time of the invitation from MWTH, I had continued to challenge every sign of pressure to offer bribes to the detriment of neonates. I strongly believed that the idea of offering or asking for bribe as a condition when the life of a baby was at stake was immoral, heartless and unethical, as well as a social injustice against these tiny members of the human race. I vowed to quit rather than join in this evil.

My continued success, despite all the opposition from covetous hospital staff, motivated me all the more to pursue this truth. I was now beginning to express my displeasure to anyone whose behaviour suggested they would put financial gratification over the lives of the babies for which I had travelled so many miles, criss-crossing the entire country.

Dr Stune, the consultant clinician in charge of the SCBU, took me to the CMD's office for this meeting. The CMD, Professor Nahosuwa, was a well-built, tall and elegant man. He welcomed me and offered me a seat.

'I have heard so much about you and the great job you are doing repairing baby incubators,' he said. 'I understand you have achieved the same success at a number of hospitals and we wonder if you can also help us here. Dr Stune must have shown you our incubators, I guess.'

'Sure, I can do my best for your hospital,' I said. 'This is the reason I honoured your invitation, sir.'

'We need to be convinced that you are able to fix our incubators, so I will give approval for you to be issued a jobbing order to re-programme one of them,' said the CMD. 'We may call for more if you satisfy my doctors on the first job.'

Unknown to me, Professor Nahosuwa was beginning to work out how he might use me to his advantage. But he sounded impressive, so I did not delay scheduling the Isoko job for execution. After a few days of clinical and technical trials of the repaired incubator, there was no delay in the payment process, and a couple of months later Professor Nahosuwa invited me to come for discussion on the rest of the malfunctioning incubators.

I was not prepared for what I heard next from the CMD. Professor Nahosuwa spoke some kind words about my commitment and creativity, but then suddenly he veered off and began to advise me how I should also be thinking about collaborating with influential office holders by giving them a financial interest in the venture. He continued: 'I am here today as the Chief Executive and I can give you any job – we are all young men looking for better futures for ourselves. I can give you more incubators to repair at good cost and we will jointly share the income from the business'.

The gestures, the words, the lack of sufficient sense of pity for the neonates in his speech, all set my heart boiling in anger. Standing up, I said, 'Sir, I wish to thank you for the offer but this is not the reason I came here. My mission was to see if the neonates could be helped. If I focus on these 'proceeds of business,' I might fail at the real job. Sorry sir, but I have to go now. I might return when your hospital management is ready to selflessly help these babies'.

The Professor had not seen this response coming. He stared at me, eyeball to eyeball for a moment. 'If you say so,' he replied.

'Goodbye sir,' I said, and left Professor Nahosuwa's office. As I journeyed home, I thought of the events that had unfolded in the last two hours. I was proud of myself for being able to stand my ground before that 'big man'. I wondered where the boldness had come from to talk to him like that. If I continued with this approach, would I still be relevant? Wouldn't they gang up against me? But why should such a high-ranking officer be so bold to say such a thing against these neonates? How much money did he want to make before he could take pity on them for what they were suffering? Why should such a high-ranking executive put his personal interest above the lives of these poor tiny babies? So I kept pondering as I drove in disappointment back to Owerri.

Buisi the neonatologist

I was not alone in feeling heartbroken on seeing endless neonates being wrapped in tiny cartons and boxes to be taken away for burial. One of my old trainees on the Paediatrics Incubation Technique course at Eastern Teaching Hospital Asaba in 1997 was now consultant in charge of the SCBU at the Umuahia Federal Infirmary (UFI). Dr Buisi was a born neonatologist with great compassion for neonates, and he had worked hard to try to end the high mortality rate in Umuahia. He succeeded in persuading the management of his hospital to bring me to help. I was able to re-programme a number of their incubators, working alongside Dr Buisi, who had become a very close friend of mine.

We shared our dream of ending the era of high neonatal deaths. I had observed on several occasions that when a baby died, Buisi would stand in a corner wiping tears from his eyes because the baby had lost its battle for life. Dr Buisi worked with his science, his mind and his compassion; he was a great friend of the neonates. For people like him, there was no acceptable reason why Nigerian neonates should die at such a high rate.

The survival rate at the Umuahia centre greatly improved following the repair of the incubators, and nurses and doctors were very happy at this. Buisi worked hard to establish a signed contractual agreement between the hospital and Pokaiz Engineering Limited. This lasted for some years, but when another CMD who sought gratification assumed office, things changed. I was uncompromising, and eventually I had to withdraw my consultancy from the hospital. The poor neonates were left to whatever the in-house technicians could do for them. Such desperate money-seeking CMDs were still being appointed, knowingly or unknowingly. Their appointment was another reason why Nigeria neonates died.

Accreditation

The regulators of postgraduate medical education in Nigeria mandatorily re-assessed the quality of training and clinical practice periodically at tertiary hospitals in order to renew their training licences. This was called accreditation. Every department of a tertiary hospital that had resident doctors training to become consultants in their various fields of medicine had to prepare to face the national or West African accreditation team assigned to assess them at a scheduled time.

Dr Buisi told me that the restoration of the functional capacities of his incubators and the staff training courses that followed were huge steps forward in his desire to build confidence in his hospital for residency training in Paediatrics. The Umuahia hospital was beginning to employ more doctors and nurses in Paediatrics and Buisi had told the CMD: 'It is important, sir, by my personal conviction, that we improve the quality of our practice tools and hence general care at my department. It is very important to me that my patients get the best care to survive. Other things, such as postgraduate training, are desirable, but my primary concern is the care we presently give'.

I had already discovered that most senior consultants and heads of departments and medical directors in Nigerian hospitals were not as persuasive and passionate as Buisi. Dr Buisi was extraordinary. Many other executives I had met were hardly bothered about increasingly high infant and neonatal mortalities at the centres. They hardly scrutinised the review of mortality cases, so patients continued to die of similar causes. It was a well-known fact in Nigeria that the CMDs operated these tertiary hospitals with meagre funding and resources, so those appointing them ought to carefully assess their abilities and economic management skills. Unfortunately many of them were disastrous in the area of economic management of resources. They only seemed to learn on the job – after appointment – how to prioritise in low-funding situations. Perhaps there needed to be conscious earlier appointments geared at coaching would-be Chief Medical Directors.

No thanks to the obvious lack of these prerequisites, many of these CMDs completely forgot that the SCBU patients – the neonates – were humans, not rats or rabbits. This was why a hospital with a SCBU of 40 cot spaces would run for over five years without a single functional incubator, irrespective of rising neonatal deaths. Countless unfortunate babies were being sent to untimely graves.

Lack of the necessary equipment could not motivate good clinical practice. Managers of hospital funds would not bother to listen to words of reasons such as Dr Buisi would give, year in year out. The poor parents of these neonates could not seek redress at courts of justice or even some kind of journalistic exposure of these undesirable acts of tertiary hospital managers. Many of them were illiterates, naïve and timid, accepting all the 'cover-up' reasons the doctors gave them. Managers saw the regular packing of neonates in paper boxes out of the SCBU for burial; they heard and saw the regular heart-wrenching walling of the mothers of deceased neonates; they saw the heartbroken fathers and clinicians like Buisi wiping the tears from their eyes; yet they were never moved to do something about it. Some Nigerian hospital workers, sadly, were happy so long as their salaries were coming in month by month, and bribe money was coming too, contract after contract. They would not mourn when the neonates died; they would not fight when neonatal mortality was rising; they would not carry placards at the entrance gates of the management buildings when paper boxes

carrying dead neonates were being taken out of the hospitals –
no, they were not bothered. If a parent dared to take pictures of
the broken-down and dilapidated hospital infrastructure, their
cameras were seized and they were harassed by the security
men for taking such information without permission. When did
these hospital workers ever cry out over such a bad situation?
When did they carry placards? When did they seek to speak to
journalists? When did they complain to the public against their
managers? You know the answer as well as I do – only when
their salaries were delayed or not paid in full!

By the way, I had often asked colleagues who cared to listen
how much a baby costs if put in monetary terms by their value
system – "Is this much less than a staff member's salary?" What
could ever move the hospital manager to remember that SCBUs
should be functional? Accreditation? Yes, that mattered more
to them than a baby's life! This is because if they failed to pass
paediatrics accreditation due to a poor SCBU, the newspapers
could report it and they might become unpopular and their
management skills criticised; they might even get queries from
their government employers.

One evening, Dr Kumara of MTH Mbong called me to tell
me that Dr Etenora, head of department at Igwocha Tertiary
Hospital (IGTH) in Port Harcourt, wanted me to assist
them. They had no functional incubators and the date was
fast approaching when a team of doctors from the National
Postgraduate Medical College would begin assessment of
their department for accreditation. Failure could lead to
the withdrawal of their training licence. Hence, the hospital
management were worried and wanted a swift intervention to

get the incubators working. Dr Etenora was worried that they might fail accreditation without functional incubators. Perhaps their CMD had instructed her to get someone to fix the systems before the accreditation team arrived.

I contacted Dr Etenora and later visited her SCBU at the IGTH. As the doctor showed me round, she explained that the situation had remained the same for over five years, leading to soaring neonatal mortality. I was sad that it had to take so-called 'accreditation' for this big teaching hospital to think of the SCBU when they had done nothing while all the 12 incubators I saw had broken down, one after another, until none remained to save the neonates with. I wished I could refuse to help them, so that they could fail this accreditation and face the shame.

After observations and all assessments, I was finally taken to the CMD, Dr Egenetus. The CMD's deputy, popularly known by the title of Chairman Medical Advisory Committee (CMAC), Professor Goodman Itaro, was passionate about the survival of neonates, and he accompanied me and Dr Etenora to the CMD's office. Dr Egenetus was a huge man with intimidating structure, a deep voice and a look in his eyes that could frighten anyone.

At the end of the meeting, I promised the CMD and his colleagues: 'I should be able to get seven of these systems working before the stated accreditation date. However, I have had ugly experiences of hospital management slowness in settling my bills after work. I also figured out that this undeserving punishment I suffered was because I refused to honour several individuals who made inappropriate demands from me. I hope it would not be the same here, because I will fight back'.

'Your money will be paid as soon as your job is certified to have been satisfactorily completed,' said the CMD. 'We do not delay payments in this hospital, all right?'

A Jobbing Order was issued and the work was completed, tested and certified by the user department and the SCBU. This was achieved ahead of schedule, eight days before the accreditation start date. My bill was submitted to the CMD for his approval for the bill to be processed for payment. The doctors and nurses of the IGTH SCBU were very happy with the great job I had done, and many of them did not hesitate to show their personal appreciation. Amongst these was the ward manager of the SCBU, Mrs Aroma, who began to pray for me, saying: 'The Lord will bless you and make you prosper in this your passion for the neglected neonates'. She continued, 'After many years of nursing practice, I am so thrilled to see an engineer with such a passion for neonatal survival. The god of the neonates will continue to protect you and you will mount heights in your career'.

I was gladdened by this gesture and felt I could look forward to many more years of working with this particular centre to help improve neonatal care practice. But I might have been wrong in thinking that everyone at the hospital appreciated my hard work. I returned after six days, as I reasoned that my cheque must be ready for collection. I went to the cashier's office only to find that my payment file had not even reached the Accounts Department, let alone been processed for payment. It had to go through the Director of Administration (DA) and various desks in his office before being returned back to the CMD for final approval based on any administrative recommendations before proceeding to the Accounts Department.

'You may go and find out where exactly your file is at the moment, then discuss with the officer in possession of the file at the moment in order to push it to the next desk,' said the cashier.

What a pile of crap, I thought. 'You know what,' I said to the cashier, 'I am not prepared for this nonsense.' I walked away. I was now boiling inside, thinking that this was exactly how they had pushed the neonates to the back seat in their prioritisations. I thought what a pleasant surprise it would have been to get to IGTH and find my cheque ready for collection. However, I had already worked out what my plan B would be if they attempted to mess with me. I went in to see the CMD, but was told he was too busy to see visitors. I became impatient and left Dr Egenetus's office. I was determined to fight for the neonates. I would teach these heartless adults a lesson that would make them ever remember the neonates.

I went straight to the SCBU, detached the power-pack modules from all the re-programmed incubators and locked them in the boot of my car, which was parked outside the SCBU building. The Ward Manager (matron in charge), Mrs Aroma, was unsuspecting, as she thought it was part of the check-up procedure. I went back into the SCBU and told the matron that I was going back to Owerri with all the removed modules until the hospital paid the bill.

'Oh, but our accreditation starts tomorrow, did you tell the HOD and CMAC?' asked the matron.

'I came here to work for the survival of the neonates and not for the pleasure of the accreditation team,' I replied. 'What's more, I don't have any business talking to the tricksters who could not keep their promises of payment within three days of completion,' I angrily replied and left for my car.

As I was about to drive off, the matron hurried to her telephone, called the HOD and CMAC, and reported the incident. The CMAC quickly issued instructions to the exit gate security post and before I could reach the exit, the security officers had shut the gate. I stopped my car in the middle of the road with three other cars ahead of me. Within a few minutes, the CMAC and HOD arrived and began to plead with me to return the removed modules for the sake of the accreditation that was to start the very next morning.

I turned my engine off and refused to move my car. I asked for my money to be brought to me before I would listen to anyone. Then the news reached the CMD of the chaos going on at the exit gate. He sent a messenger to ask the CMAC to come along with me to his office to collect my cheque, but I refused to move, demanding that cash be brought to me at the gate instead of a cheque. 'I no longer believe any of your words,' I said. 'How can I be sure your cheque will not bounce at the bank?'

Dr Egenetus rushed out of his office, demanded my file from the Director of Administration, and issued immediate orders to the Accounts Department to prepare a cheque. The cheque was fast-tracked and issued ahead of all the other protocols of the administrative and accounts departments. Dr Egenetus was then driven to the gate in the company of a man from the cash office with the cheque and a 'collections register' to be signed by me. The CMAC and the HOD stayed at the gate with me for over two hours before the CMD arrived. I agreed to go with the cashier to the bank to pay in the cheque whilst my car remained at the gate. Payment was confirmed at the bank, and I returned and restored the modules before driving home.

I wondered why it had taken the fear of failing an accreditation assessment to make them provide essential life support for the neonates. Why did neonatal life seem so low in value in the eyes of these administrators? When accreditation was over and they had their pass mark, would they ever remember the neonates until the next accreditation years hence?

Trade Unions against the neonates

For the record, it must be said that I had high respect and regard for a good number of the doctors and nurses that worked in the Nigerian SCBUs. In an interview a few years later, I said:

'During strike action for non-payment or insufficient payment of salaries and emoluments, when union members forcibly removed every worker from the hospital premises in protest, many of my comrades would sneak into the SCBUs, especially the nurses, and in distressing situations they would continue to battle for the survival of the neonates. God bless these kind-hearted ones. How I adored them! But they were hardly appreciated by the hospital management, who would later take the glory for any minimal successes achieved during such times. They were regularly victimised through non-payment of 'overtime' money due to them or appropriate promotions when due. They were often ignored when they complained of lack of appropriate tools for their work, often intimidated with such comments and questions as: 'The SCBU does not generate any meaningful money from the practice;

where should the money for your demands come from?' In spite of all these provocations, many of these comrades never gave up. The administrative notion that SCBU generated little or no revenues and must stop asking for too much got so bad in years to follow that some CMDs adopted a draconian rule of executing needs of various departments based on the amount of internally-generated revenue coming from their units. This created a huge imbalance, including neglect of the neonatal wards that couldn't measure up to other adult departments, and hence led to even higher mortality. Why must such bad rules be put in place against these poor innocent neonates?'

The paediatric doctors had often been unable to counter this argument because many Nigerian men cared little about sick new-born babies and would not want to 'waste' their money on a tiny patient when they were unsure of its survival. I felt helpless to argue as some doctors still looked down on me as being professionally inferior.

I may wage a war for the neonates against these known enemies within the rank and file of hospital and government bureaucrats, but what do you do when the babies' own parents turn out to be the reasons why they died? It was a Tuesday morning in one of my busiest SCBUs in the north of Nigeria. I was inside the ward and heard angry voices and noises coming from the nurses' station. It was unsual, so I went out to investigate. There was the ward manager, a crying nursing mother and a group of three men furiously arguing.

'Is there any reason why the differences may not be settled in a lower tone, Matron?' I asked. Pointing at one of the men, the matron replied, 'This man is Mr Isama, the father of the 750g neonate in incubator bay No.12. He came here insisting on taking away the baby, but I advised him that the baby will not survive if discharged now'.

I needed a three-stage interpretation chain to communicate with the man as he neither spoke Hausa language nor English. The matron understood Hausa and English but not the man's tribal language. It was a long process, but the neonate needed help without delay. I engaged with the man, requesting that he allowed us to take care of the child and explaining that the baby could not survive outside the incubator, not even for 48 hours.

'This child has been here for eight days and I don't have the money to pay for the hospital bills, hence I want to take the baby away,' said Mr Isama.

'Okay, in that case, I can assist you to pay the infant's bill, just allow the baby to get stronger before taking him away,' I said.

'I will then go with my wife. We can come back after one week to take him from the hospital,' said the man.

'No, this is not possible as we need your wife around to produce milk for us to feed your baby.'

The man insisted that he had no money to provide for his wife staying behind at the hospital with the child. It was clear to me that going by the neonate's situation, there was almost no chance of survival outside the incubator; hence, I decided to extend my offer to the man.

'I will pay for your wife's stay, only let her alone to produce milk for feeding her baby,' I said. The interpretation got to the man but it was now taking long for my chain of interpreters to give me feedback. I could notice arguments and dialogue between the man and the kinsman who was translating to

Hausa. Meanwhile the nursing mother was increasing her heart-wrenching sobbing.

'What's going on, matron? Why aren't they saying anything to me?' I said. Just then the interpreter began to speak to the ward manager. 'I don't want anything that will keep my wife behind. I can 'dash' you the child if you like; you can take him, but I want to go now with my wife,' said Mr Isama.

'But what about the mother, what does she want?' I asked the matron.

'The woman's wish is irrelevant as whatever the man decides goes. The woman wants the best for her baby but the man will not let her stay,' said the matron. This was how the man took the poor neonate away to whatever fate might befall it.

Situations like this and attitudes such as that displayed by Mr Isama were regular issues that hardly ever came into the open to be condemned and criminalised by the wider public. The nursing mothers were subdued to quietly carry the burden whilst burying their babies, just because the men could pin them down soon after to produce more babies unhindered. Such cases were clinically concluded in the admission register as 'discharged against medical advice (DAMA)'. The clinician is exonerated so long as DAMA has been written against the case. DAMA can often be seen in registers, but how much does the public know the atrocities behind these cases. How many people have been prosecuted for 'unlawful' DAMA?

It was now obvious to me that the battle for neonatal survival had many fronts and if it was to be won, they must all be attacked. I had been confronted with many reasons why the neonates were dying. I continued to study all situations, but the frustrations and discouragements were endless. What about the future, I wondered? How could I still remain relevant for these neonates in ten years' time? Yes, there had been reasonable successes across the country but none came without unpredictable non-clinical battles rooted in the insatiability of administrators, technicians and the public. Indeed, non-clinical or non-nursing activities were contributing huge amounts to the reasons why they died.

My worries continued, but the event that would force me to change my strategy for the future was yet to unfold.

CHAPTER 5

THE MDG4 RACE

✦✦✦✦✦✦✦

All the initial contacts, conference exposure and demand for my interventions clearly confirmed to me that the neonatal aspect of MDG4 was a crucial part of the Millennium Development Goals which had to be decisively controlled for Nigeria to achieve the target. Dr Kumara of MTH Mbong had earlier informed me that by his practice perception, the death rate of newborn babies was far higher in comparison with the death rate of the whole under-five cohort, yet little was being done about it. He informed me that many factors were responsible, of which the lack of functional incubators was among the greatest, if not the greatest.

This information was confirmed a few months later when Professor Norman of Asaba hospital invited me to tackle their broken-down incubators. All professional contacts, now fast growing in number across tertiary hospitals in Nigeria, seemed to emphasise that they lacked adequate functional incubators and without them they perceived that Nigeria could not make reasonable progress. However, none of them could provide me with the actual quantification of this lack in terms of its fractional contribution towards the death rate of under-fives. One message was quite clear though, and this was that incubator intervention was a crucial factor that must be tackled in the MDG4 race.

I went back to sourcing as many journal publications as I could find in order to read more on this subject as related to Nigeria. I soon realised that a number of publications from Nigerian authors agreed with all I had heard from Kumara, Norman and the other paediatricians who cared to relate with me. I could identify arguable lapses in some of the articles, but I still lacked what Nigerians perceived as the 'clinical or academic' qualifications I required in order to join in the argument. They cared more about academic qualifications and the countries/institutions where these were obtained from rather than the sense in the argument.

Many articles I read identified the problems, but none provided solutions. Why weren't they engaged with developing a local solution, I wondered? Why must the solution be based on importation of ideas and devices that I had seen littered everywhere – devices that could not even be maintained? Neonatal incubator intervention must be fully understood, as this seemed to be much more than having a box that generated some heat.

I began to question what incubator functionality, measurement of efficacy and best practices really should be. I sought to know what alternatives there might be to this complicated machine, if it was so important for the survival of this precious class of humans. I read widely and consulted the few paediatrician friends I had made across the country. All these friends contributed immensely to an initial neonatal education that would propel me into asking many more daunting questions.

One of those early great friends was Dr Sump at the SCBU of Jos Teaching Hospital. I reasoned with Sump and the others that accepted me and often deliberated on how systems were being affected by factors such as power supply, humidity and lack of human manipulative skills for effective incubator control. I had little clinical understanding of neonatal anatomy and physiology. However, I perceived that many factors associated with neonatal thermal requirement other than the incubator itself might be making negative contributions in the Nigerian setting, but what could these be? A lot needed to be understood in Nigerian cultural and economic terms, perhaps, in order to win this battle. Could there be a better neonatal outcome in some kind of 'unconventional' incubator technique tailored specifically to address the Nigerian setting? What could be done differently to achieve this? Should they resort to some kind of indigenous tweak that could specifically address some of the peculiar factors identified locally?

Polite brand neonatal systems

In 1998, I decided to design and launch PEL's own brand of neonatal systems in order to establish the company as a major player in the country's race towards the MDG4 target. The prototypes of the systems were completed and ready to commence clinical testing by the third quarter of 1999. I reasoned that this must, however, be preceded by two important groups of assessors I must invite – engineering professionals and medical professionals. The Nigerian engineers were the first to visit, led by the President of the Nigerian Society of Engineers, and shortly followed on another day by the Nigerian paediatricians, led by the Chairman of the Paediatrics Division of the National Post Graduate Medical College of Nigeria.

The engineers were pleased with the standards and quality of the fabricated systems. After a couple of technical questions, observations and suggestions by the team, the President summarized the impression of the team in a document that stated: 'This visit is an eye opener. The achievement of this centre is a good testimony to what Nigerian engineers can do, given vital support. There should be a presentation of the equipment to the nation.' Similarly in a write-up on behalf of the visiting team of paediatricians, Professor Azubuike wrote: 'I remain impressed by the products of your company. I am happy to confirm that my initial impressions of Engineer Hippolite remain unchanged. Please keep it up'.

The various observations were noted and used to validate the final prototype for use. Thus, the systems were commissioned to begin clinical testing at the Federal Medical Centre, Owerri.

My fame amongst my chartered engineer peers at the Nigerian Society of Engineers (NSE) soared. I was decorated that same year with the prestigious Presidential Merit Award of the Engineering Society for my contributions to engineering development and my services for the survival of Nigerian neonates at a ceremony in the city of Ilorin themed 'the Pankeke nite'. The president and deputy president of the NSE were particularly pleased with the high respect my work was bringing to the Engineering Society. They pledged to assist in whatever way they could to ensure that my work among the Nigerian neonates could be progressed.

I might have acquired a lot of technical experience to be of help to the neonates, but my deep desire was to also investigate other compelling factors, in addition to providing reliable machines. There was a problem here though – many doctors seemed reluctant to pay attention to whatever medical discovery I might make, because I was 'just an engineer' and not someone with a formal academic training in a medical subject. This was my feeling based on the treatment I received whenever clinical issues were discussed. If I was to satisfy my passion to help the dying babies and feel truly empowered in making acceptable discoveries for them, a huge sacrifice might have to be made. I would have to attend a medical school of some sort for formal academic training on the basics of medicine; I would have to master human anatomy and physiology and find a way of driving engineering-biased medical research on neonatal survival. I would not opt for any low-class university for this; it had to be the best, or one of the best, in the world. I was tired of being made to feel inferior by snooty questions such as 'where were you trained?' This strategy was the only way to go to earn the respect of snobbish professionals in such a nation that adores certificates, with or without practical substance. The question however remained how this could be actualised, and where the funding for the required foreign currency could come from. So I faced a puzzle. It was like a mountain to climb before I could see the dawn of my dream day.

A 'biblical Job'!

My plans for further study relied on foreign universities, but this looked impossible as I could not make enough money from my job to fund it. I made initial attempts to gain a Commonwealth scholarship, but failed because I had no one to bribe assessors for me – a Nigerian issue. I began to feel there was no point in dwelling on this impossible dream. I had no one to help me, family, friends, colleagues or government. Perhaps I would be better giving up all these crazy fantasies and putting myself forward for employment in the booming oil and gas industry. However, I was not sure if giving up was the right way to go. I would quickly recall all the difficulties I had already met in my career so far. I also remembered the successes I had achieved without any help from the individuals and organisations which I considered should have helped. One after another, all my past experiences were rolling by in my mind like a movie.

And then came the memory of a nightmarish event which nearly claimed my life. It was classical, it was brutal, and it exposed the extreme wickedness of some Nigerian civil servants.

It was still early in my career. My medical laboratory systems were creating waves across Nigeria. The different models of my laboratory incubators, centrifuges, waterbaths, etc. were being marketed by a number of vendors. I came across a young dynamic laboratory reagent and equipment marketer, Ambutu, formally based in the northern city of Jalingo but in the process of relocating his business to eastern Nigeria. Ambutu was very pleased with my skills and soon linked me up with Dr Okeaki, a State Commissioner of Health from Benue State in the Nigerian middle-belt region. At the time, Dr Okeaki was frantically searching for a capable professional to assist in fixing numerous items of laboratory equipment that had broken down at his State-owned General Hospital (SGH). Dr Okeaki quickly invited the relevant Ministry of Health staff to his office to introduce them to me. A good number of these were staff of the SGH. Two top State Ministry of Health (SMoH) staff, namely the Director General (DG) of the Ministry, Mr Kwale, and the Director of Hospital Services, Dr Oganude, were also invited.

The Commissioner allowed Mr Ambutu to make a presentation on what he knew about my laboratory equipment capabilities and designs. Ambutu did a good job and I could see happy looks on the faces of those present; for me this signalled satisfaction and approval'.

After patiently listening to my own presentation, the Commissioner was fully persuaded that I was capable of handling the SGH job. I went ahead to demonstrate how I could recover most of the State's abandoned laboratory systems across the local government areas, if given the opportunity to do so. The meeting ended with the Commissioner detailing Mr Kwale, the Director-General, to award a contract for the restoration of the broken-down laboratory equipment at the SGH to me, and directing him to make all necessary arrangements to ensure that my payment was not delayed upon completion of work.

I liaised with the SGH staff to identify about 19 different systems to be repaired in the first phase of the project. This initial job was calculated to cost a total of ₦147,000.00 (the equivalent of US$23,363 at the time). Some of the top hospital staff approached me to inflate the cost of these repairs in order to create room for their own 'cut' of the income. As usual, I turned down the private requests of the SGH staff to inflate the cost in order to accommodate their interest; this made their enthusiasm for the job diminish. They would have frustrated the submission of my contract quotation to the SMoH but for the involvement of the Honourable Commissioner, who wanted to see this job executed without delay. Surprisingly, Mr Kwale, the Director General, also exhibited the same moves and made advances to me for the inflation of the cost, but he was ignored too. I had made more enemies than I could handle, even before a contract letter was given to him. It was not obvious to me how horrified the civil servants had been by my righteous stance. They were unhappy with me, but even so, they all obeyed the Commissioner by awarding the contract.

However, unknown to me, they had a bigger plan. They were determined to crush me for daring to be so idealistic. I asked the SMoH to pay me some money upfront as a mobilisation fee to get started. Mr Kwale, full of evil plans, deceitfully responded: 'This will not be possible immediately; however, I can assure you that your payment will not be delayed once you finish the job. You may borrow money from a bank or any source, since your immediate payment is guaranteed. You heard the Commissioner say so, did't you?'

Mr Kwale was a well-built man, very elegant and looking respectfully responsible on the outside. But on the inside he was probably the opposite. I did not suspect that he could be planning evil against him.

I completed the job and handed the restored laboratory machines over to the SGH staff, and these were immediately re-engaged at work. My nightmare was about to begin. I submitted my request for payment, but for over eight weeks following this Mr Kwale gave excuse upon excuse for why my papers had not been processed for payment. I made several journeys from Owerri to the middle-belt city of Makurdi, at least once every two weeks, to plead with Mr Kwale to honour his promises to pay my bill. All my efforts failed.

The Director of Hospital Services of the State MoH, Dr Oganude, was a humble, soft-spoken man, the opposite of Mr Kwale. He pretty much sympathised with me as he tried to find out why Mr Kwale seemed to be unwilling to facilitate the payment. I later learnt that Mr Kwale's actions were a typical move to compel me to negotiate a cut or bribe for him and the other interested staff. For this man, there was nothing wrong in withholding the payment and endangering my fragile future with the unpaid bank loan I had got to execute the job. Nothing would keep Kwale from getting his share of the money owed to me.

However, I would never give in. I would bluntly say: 'No sir, I don't do such things'. I also maintained my stance when Ambutu and others dared to advise me to negotiate a cut with Kwale. I was righteously stubborn.

The Commissioner learnt about all this, and being aware of what could be going on, he tried to intervene. Mr Kwale moved quickly and connived with the other bribe-seekers, replying to the Commissioner: 'The payment papers have not been processed because not all the repaired machines are actually working properly. It might be good to advise Mr Hippolite to come and sit down with us to discuss this job and resolve the terms.'

I was outraged, as this was the first time I had heard this claim. In fact the laboratory machines had been put to work every day for over eight weeks since they had been fixed. The Commissioner wanted to advise me to go to a private meeting to negotiate with them, but I had a different plan. Everyone was still expecting a 'yes' answer, until I paused, thinking. I raised my head and looking at each of my accusers and the Commissioner watching keenly, I asked them: 'What if some systems are actually working well; will you pay for these?'

'Yes, of course,' quickly responded Mr Kwale as the Commissioner listened.

'Okay then,' I responded: 'In that case, can your laboratory staff here look through this list and indicate the systems they believe are working perfectly?'

I handed the list of the repaired items over to the Commissioner. 'Just put a tick on the functioning items,' said the Honourable Commissioner as he handed the list over to the Chief Laboratory Officer.

They consulted and indicated only eight systems out of the 19 repaired systems, hoping that I had been put in a really tight corner. I was disappointed, but I had already had enough of these crooks. Turning to the Commissioner, I said: 'Sir, this is a really bad thing to happen to me, that these fellows used the systems I repaired for over twelve weeks and ended up with such a claim as this, probably to achieve some personal aims I may not understand. This job took me ten days to finish, but for the past three months I have been so ill-treated. Since I have now lost my confidence in their honesty towards this job, I wholeheartedly accept this verdict with no further questions. I plead for the cost of the accepted eight pieces of equipment to be paid to me without further delay. I wish to give up doing any more work on these systems. I am also happy to forfeit the costs I incurred fixing them, as I can no longer stand the ugly tendencies that have been exerted upon me right from the inception of this project.' Raising my hands up, I added: 'Thank you, Honourable Commissioner. I give up, sir.'

The Commissioner pleaded with me to change my decision and fix the 'misunderstanding' with the civil servants, but I refused and insisted that it was all over. This was not the kind of answer the men had anticipated, but they would be condemned if they rejected it. So Mr Kwale said: 'Fine, that's okay. So we have to process the papers for the payment of the cost of the eight systems.'

'When do I come back for my cheque then?' I asked.

'You need to allow us up to one week for this to be ready,' answered Mr Kwale.

They all rose up and left the Commissioner's office.

Mr Kwale, however, refused to keep his promise of paying for the eight systems within a week. The Commissioner signed approval for immediate payment on the same day of the meeting, but Mr Kwale and his men dumped the papers. I realised this only a week later when I returned to Makurdi to pick up my cheque. I had seen some dishonest people in Nigeria, but never at the level of wickedness shown by some of the people I had met here.

I made two further trips over the following two months to meet Mr Kwale for my payment, but received nothing. It had become a deliberate act of victimisation, as Mr Kwale continued to give me appointments and fail to meet them. It never bothered him that it was a six-hour journey in each direction and that I was often forced to sleep overnight as I could not catch the last public transport leaving the motor parks for the east. The costs of the journeys continued to mount, thereby bringing endless frustration to me.

Meanwhile the friendship between Dr Oganude and me grew as we discovered that we had something in common – we were both Pentecostal Christians. We both believed it was not necessary to take revenge against oppressors like Mr Kwale; God was the undisputable avenger of all evils and the defender of the oppressed.

One more time, seven months after the completion of the job, Mr Kwale disappointed me again after asking me to come to Makurdi for my cheque. Bewildered by his meanness, I said: 'Sir, I never believed you were capable of doing all this to me, going by your kind comments on the very first day I met you at the Commissioner's office. Now you have become so unfriendly to me, with all kinds of dread running through my nerves whenever I come here to plead for my payment. Please sir, tell me that you do not want to pay me, and I will stop coming.'

'Oh, that is not the issue,' Mr Kwale said. 'Come in two weeks and I will make sure your cheque is ready for collection.'

I left the man's office and headed for the motor park, hoping to catch late transport. It was still only about 5 pm, so I decided to commence my six-hour journey back to Owerri as I did not have enough money to pay for hotel accommodation at Makurdi. No direct vehicle links Makurdi and Owerri, so the journey was normally made with a change-over at the city of Enugu.

I got to Gariki Motor Park in the city of Enugu at about 8.30 pm and boarded another vehicle for the last lap of the journey back home. It was night time, but the driver of the car said not to worry as he was going to drive carefully. Despite this, an hour into the journey the car had a near-miss head-on collision with a lorry on the highway at about 10 pm. I was the only passenger in the car. The driver was quick to swerve into the bush as he tried to avoid the fast-moving lorry, which was in the wrong lane, approaching in the opposite direction. The taxi I was travelling in somersaulted twice and raced into the bush before coming to a stop.

There was silence for a moment in the pitch darkness. I momentarily lost consciousness, but then came to and realised I was still alive. Then I heard the driver say, 'are you okay?' We had both survived.

Both the taxi driver and I had sustained various injuries. Nearby villagers heard the sound of the crash and rushed into the bush in search of the victims. They had lights with them and were quite helpful. They assisted us, but I regretted ever knowing Mr Kwale.

A few days after the accident, I was coming to terms with what had happened to me. As I recovered from the shock, I began to ask myself whether there was anything to gain from all these fruitless journeys which could have prematurely claimed my life. I vowed to try again, but after this last appointment I would go no more.

On the day of the appointment, I was not very optimistic that Mr Kwale would release my money. I walked into Mr Kwale's office about noon and was greeted by his secretary. After some minutes of waiting, Mr Kwale called me into his private office.

'Good afternoon sir,' I said.

Mr Kwale responded: 'Hello, you are welcome, Mr Hippolite. I know you don't miss appointments, so I really tried to ensure your cheque was presented for signing. Unfortunately, up till now it has not been presented. I don't really know what has gone wrong. Can you go and find out why they haven't presented your cheque for signing?'

I was not prepared for any delays that would result in another night trip back home. I was devastated and disappointed once again. I replied: 'Okay sir. I will go and find out.'

During all my many visits I had got to know the various offices as Mr Kwale tossed me from one to another. I went straightaway to the Accounts Department, but was told that my cheque had not even been authorised to be written, let alone submitted for signing.

'And who is supposed to give this authorization, please?' I asked the cashier.

'The Director General,' replied the cashier.

I stared at him a while and asked further: 'You mean Mr Kwale?'

'Of course, who else would it be?' responded the cashier.

I quickly rushed back to Mr Kwale's office and told him

exactly what the accounts people had said. He replied: 'In that case you need to put pressure on them to get your cheque written by finding out and speaking to the person who is supposed to pass on your papers for authorization.' What a snake!

I had promised myself before the journey that I would be strong enough to endure any abuse Mr Kwale might end up throwing at me, and in good faith I would calmly say a final goodbye to him, irrespective of the final outcome. However, the last words from this man brought all the memories of the highway accident back into my mind. My young and innocent spirit crumbled under the weight of the cruelty unleashed by this senior civil servant. Mr Kwale was old enough to be my father.

I stood up and struggled to restrain the tears that were about to overpower me. I wiped them away and said to him in a hoarse voice: 'Sir, you may now feel free to divert this money into your own pocket as I will not come for it any longer. I narrowly escaped death the last time you asked me to come here. I think I need to apply wisdom and completely avoid any further disasters in my life. My prayer is for God to judge the punishment I suffered at your hands.'

With these words, I left Mr Kwale's office and headed for Dr Oganude's office to say goodbye to him before departing. I did my best to put on a brave face, unaware how red my eyes were. They attracted the attention of Dr Oganude, who stared at me.

'Did you cry in Mr Kwale's office?' asked Dr Oganude.

'I didn't want to, but I was unable to hold myself back,' I said, with a sob. 'I was heartbroken, but I will cope.'

Dr Oganude said: 'No, you should not have wept. This could

easily arouse God's anger against this man. God is unlikely to overlook the tears of a righteous person in this situation. I wish there was more I could do from my end, but he is my boss.'

'Okay, don't worry sir,' I said. 'Thank you for your friendship these past months. I have got to go now.'

That payment was never made. It is possible Mr Kwale and his gang eventually diverted the pay into their private pockets. However, many of them developed such reprobate minds that they never associated the calamities that befell them with the various atrocities they had committed. After all these evils, many Nigerian civil murderers such as Mr Kwale would still take the front seats in churches and mosques; they would still quote the longest bible passages and preach the longest sermons, pretending to be what they were not and could never be.

Two months after my last trip to see Mr Kwale, a fire broke out in Kwale's residence during the daytime, when everyone was out of the house. The house was completely burnt down. Nothing was rescued from the huge house and Kwale lost everything, including his university certificates, according to later stories. The source of information, one of Mr Kwale's office staff, said: 'During our condolence visit, the Director General was shaken and appeared lost in a manner I have never seen him. We prayed for him. In his response to our speeches of encouragement he said, 'I have taken everything the way God allowed it. God might have chosen to make me the biblical Job of today, the Job who lost everything he ever owned, including his university certificates.'

'Oh, give me a break!' I said in my heart. 'The biblical Job was a righteous man, but you are not.'

Indeed, Kwale could not be right, as the disastrous fire might not be unconnected with the evil he had committed against me. Dr Oganude almost prophesied that God would take revenge. It is however sad that the Nigerian civil service is full of men and women today who are many times more dangerous than Mr Kwale. He might have died a miserable man by now, but if he is still living, he is the most miserable man alive, for daring to try to end my life and hence deny the Nigerian neonates the gift of the passionate fellow I would become to them.

A very few good people like Dr Oganude do exist, but they are hardly seen or heard, sadly. I went all out to understand why these people preferred to keep quiet and do nothing. From hospital to hospital, the core reason provided for this was similar, 'to avoid being misunderstood'. What a cowardly and phoney reason to give. It was unacceptable to me. The Nigerian neonates died because good hospital staff refused to challenge dishonest behaviour affecting neonatal mortality 'for fear of being misunderstood'.

A ray of hope: the movie

As I recollected some of the horrible events that had marked the early days of my career, I realised that I could have easily been derailed. These events were so discouraging that they could have killed my ambition; however, God had still manoeuvred me through these obstacles to keep me progressing. I began to see myself more as a winner than a loser, in spite of the setbacks I had suffered. I decided to focus more on the overall progress I had made, and to use these ugly experiences to emphasise my strong character and resilience in adversity. In my new frame of mind I felt powerful, which motivated me not to give up on my plans for further studies.

Doctor Oligha was a great visionary clinician and one of the senior doctors at Umuagwo Federal Tertiary hospital (UFTH). Oligha was known for his optimism, his hard work and his great faith in the usefulness of indigenous African technology. During the early days, when I laboured to develop my designs, a man of apathy and indifference headed the UFTH. His name was Dr Kumala and he was the Chief Medical Director, while Dr Oligha was the deputy CMD. Dr Kumala represented UFTH during regional health management meetings where wide subjects of clinical interest were discussed. It was during such meetings that Dr Kumala heard about the entrepreneurial efforts of a very young Nigerian engineer who operated from a neighboring city of Owerri. Kumala sought to invite me to see him. I was excited by this, because Dr Kumala was an influential person who could support my drive for proper national recognition. Prior to this, I had, for many years, enjoyed the mentorship of a wealthy medical equipment marketer in Owerri called Mr Emeka. Emeka had made an extraordinary impact on my early career, so I had great respect for him. I also enthusiastically talked about Emeka and his contributions to my medical equipment research. Unknown to me however, Kumala bore personal grudges against two people who had separately played mentorships roles in my life. Emeka was one and the other was the director of the city's blood bank, Mrs Beatty.

I arrived at Kumala's office on time, very hopeful for an excellent meeting. Smiling, I introduced myself to Dr Kumala's secretary, who ushered me into Kumala's tasteful and beautifully-furnished office. The executive sofas glittered with purple and golden bands. It was one of the most intimidating offices I had ever entered.

'Good morning, sir,' I said to the large figure across the other side of the executive desk.

'Morning, have a seat for a while, please,' responded Kumala, pointing at the sofas.

I sat down and waited until Kumala had discharged the last person in the office. 'I guess you're Mr Hippolite,' he said, gesturing to me to take a chair at the near side of his office desk.

'Yes sir.' I nodded and sat down.

'I have heard so much about your great work during our various meetings at the Health Management Boards and I am really pleased to have you here today,' said Kumala. 'Tell me about it.'

I was happy to tell my story and explain how I believed Nigeria could be capable of great technological emancipation through the kinds of ideas I had. We spent a long time in discussion. Kumala's comments were gentle, but his tone revealed his inner surprise. He thought of the volume of achievements already recorded by this young person. He had heard about my exploits, but not to the level of detail he was now getting from me. Dr Kumala was now beginning to nurse an ambition to use this potential talent to launch a private business for himself.

He began to tell me how great my talent was and how he could make me a very rich man through a business collaboration. I certainly wanted Dr Kumala's help, but not through starting a joint business.

Dr Kumala noticed my hesitation and uncertainty. 'With all these achievements, I guess there must be someone behind you in terms of sponsorship or things like that,' Dr Kumala inquired, looking me in the eye.

I quickly told my story of mentorship and the assistance I had received from Mr Emeka and Mrs Beatty. Kumala soon realised how much I adored these two people whom he considered to be his personal enemies. He said, 'If only you can forget about Emeka and Beatty in this whole thing, I am determined to make you a rich man'.

I did not want to be a rich man if it meant abandoning my dreams of a research career, so I boldly answered Dr Kumala: 'Sir, Mr Emeka and Mrs Beatty have not gained anything from me as yet. It would be unfair to dump them after their many years of investing time and resources in my career'.

'I would not think there is any unfair play in that, because this is what life is all about, as you may soon learn,' replied Dr Kumala.

The conversation went on for some time but I was unwavering in my decision not to abandon Emeka and Mrs Beatty. Dr Kumala finally dismissed me, accusing me of lacking basic intelligence. 'I will try to describe your lack of street wisdom so that you may understand,' said Kumala. 'You are like a little child who wants to apply butter on both sides of his slice of bread but ends up soiling his hands and fingers because he fails to realise that he needs butter on only one side'.

I knew I had reached the end of the road with Dr Kumala. From then on, I would try to avoid him, since I remained aligned with his enemies.

Oligha: the excellent visionary

I had a friend in Umuagwo, an actor and a natural comedian whose name was Mr Chinwe. This was odd, as traditionally, among the Nigerian Ndi-igbo, the name 'Chinwe' is feminine. Chinwe offered to assemble a group of actors for a short drama introducing a television documentary on Nigeria's high neonatal mortality. This was aimed at showcasing the prototypes of my newly-developed neonatal systems, which were on display in the lobby of the Imo State Blood Bank, Owerri.

Mr Chinwe insisted that the premises and an ambulance from the UFTH must be used in the drama, in order to produce the effects he wanted. It was not possible to execute this project at the time, because I refused to go to Dr Kumala to ask for approval for the use of UFTH, as I felt Kumala would ensure it never happened. Moreover he was capable of rejecting the proposal, and also leaving further instructions against it even during his absence from office.

I did not tell Mr Chinwe the reason for my refusal, but insisted on waiting until Dr Kumala was away or on annual leave. The opportunity finally came when Dr Kumala was away for a week. The visionary Dr Oligha stepped in as the acting CMD during Kumala's absence. This was to be my first meeting with Dr Oligha. He warmly welcomed me to his office, although he did not at first know that this was the young engineer he had heard about.

Dr Oligha was delighted to meet me in person and promised me that he would always admire such bold endeavour by a young person like me. I quickly described my recent achievements to further impress Dr Oligha. I waited to observe the acting CMD's reactions concerning the newly-devised neonatal systems, hoping to sound him out before making any request.

Dr Oligha said, 'Hippolite, I like your strong drive and I am happy to meet you. You are the kind of young man from our state whose development this hospital must encourage. Please do not hesitate to let us know where we can help'.

'Thank you so much, sir, for the encouragement,' I enthusiastically replied.

'You are welcome, you are welcome.' Oligha nodded.

'But sir,' I continued, 'I really do have a request to make for your assistance at the moment. It concerns the new neonatal systems I just mentioned to you'. I explained the idea and the need for the drama. Without hesitation Dr Oligha signed his approval to my proposal letter, authorising the filming of the drama and the use of the hospital's facilities.

'I am afraid your CMD might be unhappy with this project, if he gets to know that this is taking place without his direct permission,' I said.

Dr Oligha reassured me. 'Why do you think so? Is the hospital his private property? The most important thing is that this is a great idea, so forget about what Dr Kumala's reaction would be.' He went ahead to add more dimensions to the drama script when I met him later with the film director, Mr Chinwe. I did not bother to tell Oligha of my encounter with Dr Kumala. The drama project was successfully executed, so Dr Oligha won a permanent place of respect in my heart. This marked the beginning of a long friendship that would last for decades and continues as this story is written.

Seven years after this event, Dr Oligha became the substantive Chief Medical Director of UFTH and did not hesitate in inviting me to initiate the hospital's incubator project in 2005. By this time, I had introduced my Recycled Incubator Technology (RIT), and had already become a popular name amongst Nigerian SCBUs. Tragically, Dr Oligha suffered a major health setback in 2006, leading to his departure from the office of CMD in 2007.

In his short time in office, Dr Oligha had displayed the same charisma that I had noted in 1996 when I had first met him. He initiated revolutionary projects at UFTH and condemned negative pressure from powerful individuals who, in the past, had connived with the previous CMDs to divert funds into their private pockets. Many of the hospital staff who aided these powerful 'bad eggs' in their actions did not like Dr Oligha's style of administration, so they sought any way of ensuring that he was pushed out of office. However his short time in office was enough for him to make huge impacts, including the revitalisation of the Special Care Baby Unit, which I helped him to achieve. His functional neonatal incubator capacity grew from nothing in 2005 to six systems by the time he handed over in 2007. Dr Oligha established my position as a Visiting Consultant at the hospital. He also participated in the research that led to my first journal publication on recycled incubator technology.

Time to go back to school

My teachings during the Paediatrics Incubation Technique courses, attended by doctors and nurses, were reported to be rich and effective. However, I fully understood that I could do better with additional formal medical training. The need to acquire better skills for medical research in order to carry out more effective scientific investigations on how temperature variations related to the stability and survival of neonates made it necessary for me to seek further academic qualifications. The best possible university, perhaps in the United Kingdom or United States of America, would be ideal.

I believed that I was being motivated by God and hence was not discouraged by my earlier challenges. My strong faith played a big role in making my dream come true. I needed divine guidance as I investigated my best university options, so I relied much on constant prayers, often with fasting. I was inspired by the attitude of the Jewish scribe, Ezra, when he had led a group of returning Jews through unknown journey, as told in the Bible, so I believed that if I constantly humbled himself before God, I would get divine guidance. Being a married man with a child to look after, I knew that my strategy must make room for many uncertainties. Within a few months of my search of the options, I decided that the best choice was the prestigious Royal University in London.

One evening I joined three other members of the Nigerian Society of Engineers outing for drinks and friendly chat at a nearby bar. At this time, I was an executive member of the Owerri branch of the society. The other members were all PhD holders and lecturers at the University of Technology, Umuagwo. I had a request to pass on to Dr Ojemba, one of the three lecturers.

'I got an email from one of your former students to pass on to you,' I said. 'It is from Ms Stella, one of the recent graduates from your Department'. I handed over the printed email to Dr Ojemba. This was a time when personal computers and emailing facilities were for only the privileged few in the society, but I had this facility in my office and was happy to assist the young lady, who at the time had married and relocated to France with her husband. Dr Ojemba read it quickly through, then laughed:

'No way! She is not the kind of academic material the Royal University accepts,' he said. 'She was bright as a student, but definitely not at the level of that prestigious institution.' Dr Ojemba looked at me. 'All right, I will write a reference for her, but I can guarantee you that the Royal won't accept her. That university is a top one in the world and for the very best academic brains only'.

I knew that Dr Ojemba had studied for his PhD at the University of Manchester in the United Kingdom, so he must know a lot about other universities there. In fact Dr Ojemba had released a piece of information that was vital to me. As I left for home later, I began to reason that if all the three PhD engineers rated Royal University so highly, it must be a wonderful place.

I read more about the University, and finally I decided to send a formal application for admission to the Department of Bioengineering. In the application letter, I narrated all my exploits in my career so far, stating my reasons for further studies. I knew little about this university at the time, but I sensed a great peace in my heart on having made the decision. I felt this peace was God's way of approving the decision.

I was filled with joy when within a month of sending my application letter, I got an invitation to join the Bioengineering

Department of Royal University to study for an MSc degree in Engineering in Medicine.

The Royal proved to be fun and strange at the same time. It was a huge challenge to be an adult student in such an intense academic environment. My preparations for departure were the most challenging tests of my resilience yet. It was absolutely necessary to embark on this journey, but the fundamental factor to enable this had not been sorted – my funding. I had no means of funding whatsoever for studying at the Royal University, from any relations, church organisations, associations or the government, despite all my efforts to communicate the need. I had to secure funding before October 2000 to be able to start my course at a cost of £26,000 (about six million Nigerian naira at that time). I had no savings. How could I fund my studies?

I shared this exciting news with my brothers, sisters, in-laws and as many well-to-do relations and friends as I could in anticipation that they would rally round me to provide the funding requirement. Everyone, both distant and close relations, responded with apparent happiness to my success, but none of them offered to help me with my vision. I would have to look elsewhere.

In the preceding year, during the annual conference of the Nigerian Society of Engineers in the city of Ilorin, I had been honoured with the distinguished national Presidential Merit Award in Engineering Excellence. I decided to cash in on my rising profile at the NSE to see if I could get some help from them. I contacted the NSE's national president, Engr. Habu, and explained my vision, requesting the support of the NSE as I solicited for funding from relevant Nigerian Ministries and

Governments. Engr. Habu gladly used his influential position as the President of the NSE. He wrote letters to the governor of my state of origin, Mr Icheku (also known as Imonaju), and three other federal government ministers, those for Health, Education and Science/Technology. In his letter, Engr. Habu introduced my impressive talents and the great advantages Nigeria could derive from supporting me to actualise this vision, particularly requesting them to help in funding my proposed programme at Royal University London.

Four months passed, but none of the Federal ministers or the Governor dared to reply to the NSE President, let alone invite me for further discussions. Engr. Habu sent reminders to the four Nigerian politicians, and one after another, with the exception of Mr Icheku, the various Ministers wrote back providing excuses for why their Ministries could not help. Engr. Habu was disappointed, particularly with the Imo State governor, who completely ignored the request and never bothered to acknowledge his letter. Unfortunately, Habu could not help me any further.

'Do these people ever bother that we are talking about dying Nigerians who could be saved through the advanced knowledge this move could bring?' I said. 'Are they bothered that many of these neonates are dying of preventable causes? An education fee of £26,000 is chickenfeed to pay to save hundreds of Nigerian lives. The Nigerian neonates are not dying for clinical reasons alone – no, these kinds of political insensitivity of government agents are more reasons why Nigerian neonates died'. These thoughts continued to overwhelm my mind.

A narrow escape from death

I began to think about the various events that had brought me to this stage. I strongly believed that God had supported me, but the events of the last couple of months had brought great doubt. Had God rejected my plans or was He simply rejecting my approach of looking all over the place for help? I had now learned to interpret what God was saying to me based on many prayers and my personal instincts. Further disappointments fuelled my doubts of ever hearing correctly from God. Although I sometimes felt I was losing my mind, I remained resolute that this whole idea was initiated by divine 'open doors', whether or not things were working out well.

When someone from the church I attended approached me with compelling information, I did not hesitate to jump at the new opportunity. This fellow informed me that the General Overseer (GO) of our African Triangle Church, the Reverend Dr Jumbo, was a good friend of the Nigerian President, Chief Usmanu Sanja. He told me: 'As a well-known traveling evangelist of our branch of the church, the GO would be happy to speak in your favour to the President, so why don't you give this a trial?'

I made several failed attempts to obtain audience with the General Overseer at his Abuja base. However, after a strongly-worded reminder to the GO in August 2000, I received an invitation. Time was ticking away and the deferment of my admission was becoming inevitable. I was now interpreting virtually every little incident as God's way of saying 'no' or 'yes'. I was always seeing God in one event and the devil in another. There was anxiety and almost perpetual frustration for me, every passing minute. I became suspicious of almost everything, as though it was defining the agents of Satan that stood against me. I often awoke wondering if I was losing my mind and becoming paranoid. How much of these day-and-night dreams were mere nightmares and how much were real messages?

I would have to keep my hard-earned appointment with the Rev. Jumbo so that the President of Nigeria himself would intervene for the neonates. I reasoned that the President could readily approve the little sum of £26,000 if he understood how much this would contribute in solving the national problem. There were countless nights of bad dreams now, but I had decided to ignore them, as I could no longer work out whether they were true warnings of danger or Satanic deceptions.

On the night of the 13th August 2000 at 7 pm, I boarded a 57-seat ABC Transport coach for the overnight journey from Owerri to Abuja to keep my appointment with the GO of the African Triangle Church. I had a strong instinct that I should not go to sleep but should stay awake and keep reading the little travel bible in my hand. I was really 'in the spirit' when suddenly in the middle of Njaba bridge, the coach crashed head-on into a haulage lorry carrying logs of wood. Both vehicles plummeted into the river with all passengers on board. After the initial bang, there was screaming and finally a deathly silence.

I thought I was dead, but then I realised that I could move my upper and lower limbs, though they were underwater. I realised that the coach had submerged tail first at an angle that left the cab above the water level. I made my way towards a window that was above the water to try to open it and escape, and as I did so I noticed a book which looked as though it had been neatly placed above the water level on one of the headrests and was completely dry. I reached it to find to my amazement that it was my little bible.

I felt a mixture of gratitude and disappointment, but began to think God must have been aware that this was going to happen. I was not giving up now. I pushed the window open and climbed out of the coach into shallow water along with one other person who had managed to get to safety. No help had arrived as yet and we were in the middle of nowhere. I could now hear many other people screaming loudly from the wreckage and concluded that there must be a spiritual dimension to this whole drama event. I was angered by these attempts by the gods or devils to destroy my life, so I went right back into the water to try to rescue the other passengers. I was helped by many other people who arrived on the scene. Every single soul was saved from the river, but the coach was a total wreck. I sustained minor injuries, but lost all my belongings except my little travel bible.

A rescue coach from ABC transport turned up four hours after the accident and took all the passengers back to Owerri, arriving at about 3.45 am. Iphii, my wife, was shaken with fear when she saw me on the doorstep of our home early that morning with plasters over my wounds. 'There was an accident,' I said as I reached out to hug my wife. The event of the last eight hours were still a nightmare and so strange to understand.

After a few hours' sleep, I woke up to the reality of the situation. I was afraid of suffering from depression and quickly had to make difficult decisions for the sake of my health. Later that evening, I called Iphii and told her that I had abandoned the whole idea of travelling to the United Kingdom and had decided to start rebuilding my career the way it had been. Although this was a difficult decision, I nevertheless felt very relieved to return to my usual work.

I wrote to a professor at Royal University to notify him of my sad decision to cancel the idea of joining them. However, in reply, the professor offered me a deferment of up to one year, in case I later changed my mind.

The disappointment never affected my love for and deep relationship with my God – Praise the Lord! It never affected my sensitivity to my instincts and inner witnesses. I still considered these events as God's ways of communicating with me, although I didn't fully understand. However, one thing I was sure of, and that was that London wasn't going to happen.

I really felt God was close to me, always communicating with me, and that I often almost heard Him clearly. None of these strange ecstasies ever made me feel weird again. I grew more confident in myself as a 'human tool' that was useful to God. I soon forgot all about Royal University and all the horrors I had experienced. I resumed my busy activities with the few hospitals and medical diagnostic laboratories I offered services to, and weeks and months passed by.

By November 2000 it had been four months since I had fully returned to my work. My normal flow of technical/maintenance visits with some of the tertiary hospitals had been resumed for many months. I now planned to start working on more contacts for the expansion and extension of my work to other hospitals. But unknown to me, God had not done yet with the neonates or forgotten my passion for their survival. In fact, He had other plans.

On the morning of 12th of November 2000, I woke with a dialogue going on in my mind. It was as if God was siting next to me asking me, 'Do you recall the cancelled Royal University move? Whose original idea was it to embark on further studies – was it yours or Mine?' I had no immediate answer as the question resonated in my mind. I tried to shrug it off, but the thoughts and the dialogue continued. The selection of Royal University London, the effortless process of securing admission and the unsolicited programme deferment – who had coordinated these, was it me or the divine providence of God? Suddenly all the extraordinary success of the events that had led to the idea of further education flooded my mind. It was clear to me that I had never engineered this whole idea, but it had been the work of God. 'And what right do you have to cancel an idea that you had never initiated?' God seemed to be asking me.

All of a sudden a strange feeling of shame engulfed me and I started to pray, apologising to God in my thoughts for making my arrogant decision without His clear permission. The dialogue was as real as if a superior being was before me, sternly interrogating me. After a while, this thought resumed and the 'voice' said to me, 'The Royal idea remains valid and must be implemented by this coming academic season. Meanwhile, get ready now and go to the tertiary hospital at the city of Igweocha. You will be offered a contract job that will be paid for without much delay as soon as you complete the job. Be careful not to tamper with the money as soon as you receive it.

You should send it all to the UK via your second eldest brother, Donald. The amount involved will be substantial enough for the first instalment of your tuition in readiness for the start of your course in October 2001'.

This was strange to me, but it was full of reality, as though I had heard someone speak clearly. It was awesome and strange, but I was filled with excitement again. It felt so real and refreshing that I was sure I was not losing my mind.

It was still only 5:30 in the morning and other people in the house were still in bed asleep. I did not hesitate to dress up in readiness for an early departure to the city of Igweocha. As soon as Iphii woke up from sleep, I told her that my plans for the day had changed. 'I felt God wanted me to go to Igweocha for a job that could pay my Royal tuition,' I said. Iphii had learned to stop questioning this talk of what God said, but she wondered aloud how this idea had suddenly been resurrected from nowhere.

Later that afternoon, after a few hours of discussions and negotiations, to my amazement, the Management of Igweocha Federal Hospital signed off a contract valued at ₦92,000 - the pound sterling equivalent of a little over £5000 – for the repair of broken-down incubators at their special care baby unit. The hospital management emphasised that the job must be completed before the approaching Christmas break. This was achieved as scheduled, and the hospital aptly paid the bill by the second week of January 2001. I packaged the money and gave it to my elder brother Donald, who was about to make a business trip to London. So my plan to go to the Royal University London was revived.

I felt very relaxed during the first quarter of 2001 as I waited for my miracle-working God to provide more jobs in order to raise the rest of the required funds, especially the tuition fee of £11,000. However, when I could not secure any more substantial work by June 2001, the pressure on me returned, crashing down on me. I nervously fought my anxiety, but my hopes were fading away again. However, I had already learnt my lesson, so I did not begin to run from pillar to post as I had the previous year. I kept calm. Whenever I slipped back into worry I managed to suppress this by recalling my 'divine encounter', especially as the first promises of that conversation had fully been fulfilled exactly. Whenever I pondered on this encounter, I felt all the more strengthened on the inside. Moreover, I was almost being haunted by that question: 'What right have you got to cancel an idea you never initiated?'

I strongly believed that another surprise would come, even if it waited until the very last minute before the commencement of my course at the end of September. The month of July was almost over when the news of the tragic loss of a baby broke out in one of Nigeria's biggest cities. This was not usually a news item, for countless neonates had died from bursting hot water bottles or had 'roasted' in malfunctioning incubators. Many such babies belonged to uneducated, uninformed or naïve parents who would normally weep, wipe away their tears and package up their dead for burial without a single question asked. There was great disrespect of neonatal lives by hospital management staff. However, on this occasion, the pattern was different. The deceased baby was related to a well-connected man, a friend of powerful people. Questions were asked, contrary to the usual expectation of the hospital management.

The mode of death of this particular newborn made this a national news item, driven by the deceased's relations to shame the hospital. There was nationwide criticism.

The incident was caused by an incubator that had been malfunctioning and causing similar tragedies for a long time. To further shame the hospital it was widely reported that the referral centre had no properly-functioning incubators, causing the deaths of many babies referred to them. It was a very difficult time for the management of the hospital, and an embarrassment to the Government, and it led to the Federal Minister of Heath making a statement on national television news concerning the tragedy. The jobs of the management staff were under threat. Individuals in the top management of the hospital had to work fast to save their jobs, so there was no hesitation in adopting any available solution without the usual prejudice or tribal bigotry.

I quickly wrote to the hospital and outlined my credentials, offering to help by restoring the incubators using my ultimate re-programming technique. The Chairman of the Hospital Management Board was particularly pleased to receive my letter and offered me an immediate contract, after verifying my technical claims. The mobilisation fee for the job was quickly paid as I demanded, and the job was completed by the last week of August 2001. The funds realised from the job was enough to take care of the balance of the Royal tuition and my personal maintenance until midway through the course.

The turbulence in my mind resumed. Should every Nigerian neonate not be treated as equally important? Why would highly-placed people close their eyes to the atrocities against babies until they were affected? This sort of state-powered discrimination was another reason why so many Nigerian neonates died. Now I was all the more determined to fight on for these poor neonates.

CHAPTER 6

A NEW LIFE IN THE UK

✦✦✦✦✦✦✦

The British High Commission at Abuja was in no hurry to process my student visa application when it was finally submitted during the first week of September. They were happy to do it at their own pace, regardless of the start date of the course. The visa was issued late, so I arrived a full month after my lectures at the Royal had started.

Dr McDaniel (later Professor McDaniel) notified me by email that I was already late for the start date as my cohort had arrived and lectures commenced. However, he added, 'every lecturer involved in your course has given a promise to offer you extra assistance provided you are able to catch up'. And so, during the last week of October 2001, I boarded a Virgin Atlantic Airways flight from Murtala Mohammed International Airport Lagos to begin a new chapter of my life at Royal University London. I had more than a month of catching up to do in a strange and sophisticated city, full of all kinds of surprises and shocks – weather, the environment, cultural shock, strange accents, technology, you name it – and the Royal University's high academic standards did not make life any easier for poor me. I was 'A' rated in written and spoken English, but the British accent was so strange and hard to comprehend initially. The great welcome I received from a friend from my teenage years, the British-born Iyke Azuka, and the clever support from Professor McDaniel were invaluable during the difficult settling-in period.

Moments came when I felt lonely, even with my busy academic schedule. I made quite a few telephone calls to Nigeria, but this could not soften how much I missed my charming and elegant wife and our energetic two-year-old daughter, Jimara. I never allowed the memories of my last night before departure to wear off; the wonderful pleasure of lying peacefully between Iphii's breasts. She was such a beauty that she could easily make any man happy, and gave such pleasure in satisfying his hunger for love and care.

I could not wait for Iphii to join me in London, but a number of hold-ups at the British High Commission in Abuja were delaying this. Mrs Johnston of the International Students Department at the Royal played a great supportive role. She never stopped communicating with BHC Abuja until finally, after six months of separation, Iphii and Jimara were able to join me at last. Little Jimara must have been very excited and expectant when she realised that she was actually going to see the father she had missed for six months.

I arrived to meet them at Heathrow airport wearing a quilted winter jacket and a strange hat – such an odd look for anyone leaving Nigeria for the first time. This was a time when cable television and mobile phone technology had not made foreign cultures such a common sight in Nigeria. Jimara stared at the strange man approaching them before she heard me call out in my characteristic way, 'Jim-B!' Then she recognised her father and ran up to jump on me.

Jimara's arrival was an emotional moment for me. I had had to go through the long process of posting a cheque by courier to Lagos in order to make up a small shortfall on her underpaid child ticket. I had wrongly expected some assistance for this small amount from one of my numerous relations residing in Lagos, or the little girl's maternal relatives, with whom they were temporarily staying. The email bombardment and demands for me to send a cheque made me wonder why my own relations could be so insensitive, unhelpful and perhaps uncomfortable with this life change for me. I wondered why no one would do it for the little toddler's sake. So I was glad that I had managed, despite all the academic pressures and my financial poverty, to get my little daughter on that flight.

We lived together at Udney Park Road, Teddington in Middlesex, and I successfully completed my research project on the function of the meniscofemoral ligaments of the tibio-femoral joint, winning the admiration of my project supervisors for my excellent approach to medical research. This project was later to win one of the finalist awards in the competition for the 2003 global best medical engineering project, organised by the

Medical Division of the Institution of Mechanical Engineers, London. My supervisors in the Bioengineering Department, feeling I had great potential, began discussions with me on the possibilities of continuing for another four years of PhD research. It had already been a huge struggle to complete the MSc programme without leaving outstanding payments to settle with Royal University, the study being entirely self-funded. The proposal by my supervisor was quite pleasing, but deep in my heart I dreaded what it might bring. I felt it was just not possible to continue my financial nightmare for another four years. But I had come here for a reason, and I had to follow my plan through for the sake of the Nigerian babies. So I provisionally accepted the PhD proposal based on two conditions – that my research would not have to be self-funded and would somehow be tailored to paediatric neonatology.

It was obvious to me that the Royal would provide many opportunities for the furtherance of medical understanding that could enhance my neonatal work. However, I could not decide whether to stay or return immediately to Nigeria. I wondered why I felt so confused. What if this was God appearing from nowhere and speaking through my supervisor? It would be disastrous to get it wrong again at this stage, and in a foreign land.

So there were many sleepless nights, and the decision was made more difficult by the fact that my supervisor was primarily a musculoskeletal researcher. A number of additional meetings were scheduled for discussions, but neither of my two conditions could be easily confirmed for various reasons. My instinct was now beginning to favour blindly opting for the PhD research for the sake of the dying neonates. During every meeting with Dr Harry, my MSc supervisor, I repeated the same question: 'Why do you want to persuade me to take up a PhD in medical research?' Time and again I got nearly the same answer. My supervisor once said, 'A PhD is not for everyone, but one of my duties is to identify and advise very talented students who have demonstrated the aptitude and ability to complete the rigorous PhD research at Royal University, and you possess such rare talents'. There was always a boost to my confidence whenever my supervisor praised the 'exceptional' research talent he had identified in me.

Dr Harry already had an orthopaedic PhD question in mind for me to tackle for the next four years. Harry did not seem to have any interest in paediatrics-related research, so I concluded that I could not work with him. I would have to seek advice from other academics within my Department.

I consulted a few senior academics in my department for advice. Professor Sotus was an admirable elderly professor of respiratory mechanics, and I would never forget the invaluable advice I received from him. I said later that Sotus had given me the best foundational research advice of my career. Sotus told me, 'Hippolite, I honestly admire the research strengths we have identified in you, but I must advise you that the PhD programme is basically a process of learning how to do research using your chosen field of study. It does not necessarily qualify you as the expert in any field, but it does prepare you with the necessary skills to become an expert in whatever field of medicine you are attracted to. Your real concern at the moment should be resolving how your study can be funded. Once that is sorted, you need one of our best young academics in the department, irrespective of his or her medical speciality, to groom you on how to carry out excellent medical research. The moment this is achieved and you are done with the research degree, you can channel the skills you learnt towards any medical passion you might have. I can advise you that if Dr Harry is willing, he is really the best person for this at the moment'.

I had hoped that Sotus would be glad to accept me as his student to begin PhD research in neonatal respiratory mechanics. Who wouldn't want a 'rocketpropelled' professor as his PhD supervisor? Professor Sotus had actually flown into space to carry out respiratory experiments on horses under zero gravity.

Although I did not get the response I had hoped for, the short lecture from Professor Sotus seemed to be all I needed to finalise my decision.

I had learnt how to flap my professional 'wings' during my early career in Nigeria, but it was Professor Harry who taught me how to soar. My relationship with Harry was that of a mother eagle and her young eaglet on training flights. It was often painful and disappointing along the way, but highly successful and profitable long-term. Harry was harsh and firm with me, but this had produced one of the world's top researchers in tropical neonatalogy; my excellence today is the attestation of Professor Harry's academic profeciency. I submitted my formal application for the PhD research with Harry as my main supervisor. 'I will learn all I can, but I will not forget the Nigerian neonates,' I promised myself as I submitted my application.

In 1992, I had attempted to seek graduate admission into Massachusetts Institute of Technology (MIT) in the United

States of America. This was after completion of my MSc degree in Nigeria. MIT required me to sit for a test in English as a Foreign Language (TOFEL). I felt there was something not quite right with that condition. I quickly wrote to MIT asking if United States English was an alien language, different from the one I had been speaking as a child and passed with credit in the West African School Certificate exams, and whether the language was different from the English I had used in submitting my Bachelor of Science (BSc) degree and Master of Science (MSc) degree dissertations at the university in Nigeria. I suggested that I did not need to take the test and would not sit for it. I posted a copy of my MSc thesis to complement my letter. My boldness and style of writing must have prompted MIT to reconsider their decision, as they quickly sent me a certificate waiving the TOFEL requirement.

I now knew that Africans are often looked upon with disdain by the self-acclaimed colonial 'masters' of the modern free world, and was determined to fight every insult against me and my race. When I had been a student at the Royal for over a year, the Royal University Registry Department sent a letter asking me to sit a TOFEL exam and to pass it before my registration for a PhD study could commence. This was to be one of the conditions for my admission to start the PhD research. What a ridiculous request, and what an insult!

I replied to the mail, referring to it as 'an insult that must never be tolerated'. I remembered how I had defended my English ability to Americans right from Nigeria, at a time when I had never travelled outside Nigeria, almost 15 years earlier. How could these fellows not give up this useless slavish mentality? I wrote, 'My successful MSc dissertation at Royal, which has been graded as well above average by your own staff, was, in fact, my third university dissertation that had been successfully submitted in English. Something must be wrong with the Royal for asking me to sit for the TOFEL exam. There must be another English language you guys speak that I am not aware of. Please explain, or I hereby refuse your demands.'

I also complained to my prospective supervisor, Dr Harry, about this insult that was absolutely unacceptable to me, notifying him of my response to the Registry Department. I also brought a copy of my old letter from MIT waiving the need to sit a TOFEL exam. 'Never mind, I will take this up,' Dr Harry replied as he tried to calm me.

A few days later, another letter arrived from the Royal Registry, advising me to ignore the earlier request. What an ugly world a poor, naïve African must live in! They push you against your rights and make unnecessary demands because they think you will be too timid to react, and you keep quiet. I learnt that I must work two or three times harder than my white counterparts in order to survive in such a hostile world with a white superiority complex.

I was the second PhD student Harry had supervised (although I became the first to graduate under him, in November 2006). The journey ahead for both Harry and I in the academic relationship was to last a difficult four years, full of disappointments and sad moments but with happy ones too. Harry's first student was Dr Matthews, a young British medic, who had started his PhD programme about six months earlier than I. My research title would be in orthopaedics biomechanics of the upper limb to investigate the functional characteristics of the glenohumeral joint ligaments. My assisting supervisor was Dr Ricky of the Biomechanics section of the Mechanical Engineering Department; hence, I became a crossover PhD student of the Orthopaedics Biomechanics section, the Bioengineering and Musculoskeletal Surgery Department.

At the first meeting, both supervisors promised to work together to secure a grant that would pay off the entire cost of the research. They were optimistic that they could obtain this within the first 15 months of my study. They hoped to obtain enough to pay for both the tuition fees and my maintenance. They promised me a research experience that would be free from funding hitches such as those I had had during my just-concluded MSc programme. I was delighted at Harry and Ricky's concerns for my welfare.

Both supervisors explained the initial things I needed to understand about the project I was about to embark upon. Dr Matthews and I worked on parallel topics related to the biomechanics of the shoulder joint, designed to complement each other. Dr Matthews soon became my friend as we battled the odds and pressures of being medical engineering PhD students at Royal University. He also had funding challenges, and Harry gave him the same promises of support to assist in securing grants for his work.

Dr Matthews was privileged, as a British citizen, to acquire a number of grants within a couple of months. This enabled him to concentrate on his studies. I had good and fulfilling inter-student research collaboration with him as our topics were closely related. However, a big gulf separated the two of us – one student had financial support from his country's institutions and the other had absolutely nothing.

When the first year was completed, I had recorded tremendous progress into the fundamentals of the research question. Harry and Ricky were both very pleased with the progress achieved; however, they had not managed to obtain any grants for me, but they continued with their promises to obtain one.

The Royal University's Accounts Department put increasing pressure on me to pay the tuition fees that had accrued. Confused, I went to Harry to inform him that I could no longer concentrate on the research as I was under immense turmoil and anguish due to this pressure. 'Ricky and I have met again to discuss over your funding and we think we should be able to get something soon,' said Harry. 'So if you can find some money somewhere to pay the Royal, we should be able to refund this as soon as we get a grant for you.'

But I had no one to turn to. The ordeals of my MSc programme had given me enough experience of neglect and abandonment by my family, relations, friends and the various arms of the government of Nigeria. I had sustained myself and my family of three by frequent trips to Nigeria to work at the few hospitals that retained me with consultancy agreements. I finally opted for the payment of the Royal fees on an instalment basis, for which I was made to sign a legally-binding document which warned me to respect the agreed payment dates. The bombardment of reminder letters for approaching or passed payment dates often made me too unsettled to concentrate on my research.

I managed to finish paying the fees despite the uncertainties of my fast-approaching MPhil to PhD transfer dissertation. I was becoming increasingly worried that Harry and Ricky might one day call me to say, 'Sorry, we can't get any grant money for you'. This thought kept coming back to my mind for many days, and it was a nightmare I would not allow to linger in my mind. I would shrug it off, feeling it would be the joke of the century if it ever happened. I refused to accept my fears that such a thing could happen, yet a deep sense of self-pity and a huge fear of rejection enveloped me. I wondered why I had had to go through all these ugly experiences in the recent past – abandoned by my own people when I needed them most, multiple bombardments from relatives, abandonment by the Christian organisations I belonged to and rejection by the government of Nigeria. A survival method must evolve. I would have to find a way of combining my compulsory full-time PhD research at the Royal with my private work in the Nigerian special care baby units, perhaps travelling to Nigeria to spend up to three weeks per trip and doing my incubator maintenance work at a few tertiary hospitals during each calendar quarter.

So I began to work out how I might establish a new strategic routine for myself. For all the years I had been away from Nigeria, I had kept my Nigerian work very active, with two technical visits every year. The few friendly Chief Medical Directors of the hospitals I visited readily paid me my consultancy fees based on the number of incubators I maintained and serviced for them, and this little income was enough to sustain me and my small family in London. My low income meant that most of our summer clothes – shoes, items of clothing and underwear for myself, my wife and child – were bought from Ariaria market in Aba whenever I travelled to Nigeria, as I could not afford to buy these items in London. I often laughed it off when people approached me during my Nigerian trips to demand gifts of clothes and shoes from London.

I made several calls to my few CMD friends concerning this dilemma. Notable amongst these was Professor Etawo. There was good encouragement from them, so I formalised a written consultancy agreement with some of the hospitals. I would have to reach out to more hospitals, as the few I had would not be enough to generate the needed funds. Some of my old friends were also rising in their career, some getting appointments as chief medical directors at other hospitals. Lasting friendships were very important to me, especially amongst my former colleagues and acquaintances.

The end of a hard-earned friendship

One of my early friends, Dr Ujonga, was promoted to the rank of professor at Okija University. He also got a position as the Chief Medical Director of Okija Teaching Hospital. Everyone expected Professor Ujonga to display the professional feats he had been known for whilst at Benin Hospital, where he had played a pivotal role in ensuring that the SCBU received my attention. Of course, it was expected that he would bring along his old friend Hippolite. The Special Care Baby Unit of the Okija hospital, where he became the overall Chief Executive, would surely be turned into the best centre in Nigeria.

I got mentally ready for this, as my friend knew all about the change he could bring to Okija SCBU, and waited until Ujonga had settled into his new job. Then, on a letter dated February 14, 2003, the invitation came. Now a UK resident and on research staff of Royal University London, I made my usual quarterly consultancy trip to Nigeria. OTH was scheduled amongst other hospitals to be visited. I would normally engage hospitals for negotiations on costing and to convince the chief executives before doing any work. Ujonga did not need to be convinced of my ability, and perhaps the financial worth of my expertise. However, I was yet to meet my worst nightmare from this axis of Nigeria.

I assessed the state of the SCBU of the Okija hospital, prepared my proforma invoice for the intended work and passed this on through to my old friend the CMD. I would normally wait for formal agreement and approval before commencement of work, but my friend assured me there was no reason to worry as the job needed to be completed before my departure back to the UK. The job was completed and after one week, I returned to see my friend and to collect my cheque. I waited in the lounge as visitors were called in to see the CMD one after another. I thought Ujonga would not delay calling me in, considering the tight schedules that characterised my short visits, but I waited a long time. At last it was my turn and I went in and sat down to see my friend. My file was brought in, but there was no payment cheque. 'Sorry, your bill has not been processed for payment as I haven't yet given approval, but I will do this now,' Professor Ujonga said.

I was disappointed and angry. 'How could you have left this undone after promising that my payment would be ready before my departure?' I said.

The CMD wrote on the file and passed this on to his office messenger to be delivered to the next processing stage. I had no intention of staying overnight in Okija that day as I had to start heading back to Lagos in readiness for my UK flight. Strangely, the CMD asked me to follow his messenger to the office where his approval for payment would be documented. I got to the next office, but was told that my payment would not be ready that week, let alone that day.

Now boiling with rage, I felt badly let down by my friend. I demanded from the secretarial staff how much had been processed for payment. 'One hundred and eighty thousand naira only has been approved, sir, you may have a look,' said the staff man. 'This is ridiculous!' I screamed. I had submitted a bill of ₦600,000 (about £1200 sterling) for the three incubators I had reprogrammed, ₦200,000 for each. The CMD had carefully avoided any negotiation, and pretended to have accepted the proforma invoice and commissioned the execution of the job. He had unilaterally slashed my bill from ₦600,000 to ₦180,000 without any recourse to his friend for cost negotiation. Ujonga had changed from an old friend who needed me to progress to the top at Benin, to an arrogant Chief Executive Officer. This was how Nigerian executives treated their very junior servants. The CMD had disregarded both his friend and, more importantly, the neonates he should have been protecting.

I was terribly disappointed as Ujonga was one person I had expected to know better. I would not have this insult! I dashed into Ujonga's office without asking permission to enter.

'What is this joke of yours?' I asked. Ujonga tried to remind me that we had known each other for a long time and the bill should have been smaller. 'That's all the more reason why you should have treated me with some respect,' I said, 'I gave you a proforma invoice and you felt too big to discuss it. You also deceived me into agreeing to work without proper negotiation. Ujonga, I completely disagree with you and you must pay my full bill.' I raised my voice in frustration.

'The hospital can't pay any more than that, I am sorry,' said the Professor.

I had no time to start exchanging words with my old friend, so I left the office. In situations like this, I would usually resort to my old tactic of doing a false ward round, where I immobilized the incubators without the immediate knowledge of the attending staff. I would normally remove a vital component specially integrated into the reprogramming setup for easy immobilization. This meant the machine would never work unless this component was restored or somehow bypassed by a knowledgeable engineer. I used this technique to compel fraudulent hospitals to pay up so that they would avoid the embarrassment that would follow. Professor Ujonga's situation would be catastrophic if this happened, as I would have left for the UK by the time the hospital realised this and made complete payment. My next visit to Nigeria would not be for three months.

I was on my way to the SCBU when it occurred to me that Chief Mika would be disappointed to hear the headline news this would cause in town. Many years earlier the elderly Chief Mika had introduced Ujonga to me, and we became friends. Over the years, Chief Mika had remained a mentor to both Ujonga and me, so he would feel disappointed that two young men he had held in high esteem were at war with each other in this manner. I wanted to be free from all blame in this matter. I would let Chief Mika know about this first, in his honour, and would immobilise the incubators afterwards.

I turned around and went to the car park. There was no public telephone at the hospital, so I had to drive to Okija town to access one. I rang Chief Mika and explained the sad situation. The Chief listened carefully. 'This is very unfortunate,' said the Chief. 'So where are you now and what do you want to do?'

'I am still in Okija, but I must immobilize the systems before leaving. I only left the hospital to pay you the respect of reporting this incident before carrying out my extreme retaliatory measure,' I said.

'When are you going back to the UK?' asked Chief Mika.

'I am leaving for Lagos tomorrow in readiness for my flight to London the following morning,' I replied.

'This is not good at all. Can I make a request from you, Hippolite? I beg that you consider not returning to carry out the immobilisation, please.'

I could not withhold my tears. 'Sir, I am not sure I can let Ujonga get away with this insult and this treatment of me,' I said, my voice cracking.

'I understand, but consider that you are building a legacy that will remain long after your working years are over. Consider the advice of an elder like me and let this situation be, for my sake and the sake of those tiny babies you are saving. Don't worry, my brother,' the Chief preached on.

'Okay, I've got to go, I got to leave this town now sir,' I said as I hung up. I left a letter of authority to pay my cheque into my bank account and left. As I drove back to Owerri, I resolved never to do any further work for OTH whilst Professor Ujonga remained the CMD. For reasons I might never know, Ujonga had destroyed a hard-earned friendship that had resulted from a shared desire to produce a solution for an extreme neonatal need, a friendship that could have saved countless babies around Okija and nearby towns. Who knew how many more needy neonates would present at this centre for the rest of the eight years Ujonga would remain the CMD? Such neonates would not benefit from what I could have done to save them. But it was all over for my work at OTH for a long time to come.

The reprogramming technique for obsolete or malfunctioning incubators had been a welcome success across many tertiary hospitals in Nigeria and had sustained neonatal thermal interventions for over seven years. But the technology was fast getting too old, as it was based on analogue (dialling knob) thermostatic input mechanism. All the broken-down semi-automatic digital systems were necessarily downgraded to the analogue technology of the reprogramming technique. I understood that there was an urgent need to look into a more modern locally-compatible electronic version for the modern age of digital controls. The need for a more efficient incubator control technology was one of the fundamental reasons for my desire to acquire some advanced foreign training. I never lost focus on this, despite my overloaded research duties in orthopaedics at the Royal.

The vast opportunities offered by its many workshops and computing facilities helped me to progress the design of a new digital system. It was often necessary to work very late into the night to keep up with the workload. I wished one thing could wait for the other. It was a mixed feeling; a digital version of the incubator solution would achieve better aesthetic appreciation and more efficient function to maintain its appeal as an acceptable alternative against the purchase of more expensive modern incubators in Nigeria. Moreover, it was sensible to make time to develop a better method of sustainability for incubator application in Nigeria, since my services were still in demand among Nigerian SCBUs.

I wanted to devise a restoration technique that could guarantee easy maintainability and operational longevity in order to minimise frequent incubator breakdown in Nigeria. I had to find a way of making these systems less dependent on the manufactures' own spare parts, which remained too expensive to purchase, and with poor supply chains in Nigeria. If neonatal survival was to improve, then incubator availability must depend on the technical ability of Nigerians and not expensive foreign engineers, I reasoned.

I strongly believed that there was no way Nigeria could meet its target on the United Nations MDG(4) standard for child survival without overcoming this deficiency, so I began to study modern interfaceable generic electronic circuits and components that could be applied to recreate a complete system whilst reusing the old casings, hoods and trolleys of the malfunctioning incubator.

I shared my proposal to develop incubator recycle technology (RIT) with my old Nigerian friend, Professor Azubuike, now an Emeritus at the National Postgraduate Medical College of Nigeria. Azubuike welcomed this as a wise idea, if it worked. The prototype of the new RIT design was installed in one of the SCBUs at Coalcity Tertiary Hospital (CCTH), with influential support from the professor. The system's technical and functionality tests were successfully completed, and the first RIT incubator began its clinical trial in July 2003 at the special care baby unit of the CCTH, one of the hospitals where Azubuike had previously worked. This was largely successful, and the news was quick to spread. The new digital system proved to be more efficient, with ease of control. The display possessed scrollable pages that could reveal useful parameters during function. These capabilities made the RIT a promising tool for extensive research in neonatal thermoneutrality. It was an extraordinary achievement for me, and within three months of the clinical trial, there was a big demand for it.

The Tertiary Hospital of Jalingo was engulfed in another incubator-related disaster, embarrassing the Nigeria Federal Government. The hospital was all out for any rescue solution, wherever it might be found. This became a great opportunity for my RIT to be applied at industrial scale for the very first time, and the ten incubator devices that had failed at THJ – representing the entire fleet at the hospital – were all restored back into service as RIT-powered systems in a two-week intervention project in November 2003. All systems were quickly subjected to an operational characterisation study as I methodologically designed, collaborating with Dr Sonpang, the young consultant in charge of the SCBU at Jalingo.

The CCTH and THJ doctors – first users of the application – confirmed that the RIT system had equal satisfactory appeal as a modern incubator but with the added advantage of being highly affordable, at only 22% of the cost of a standard modern incubator at the time. Few of my collaborating paediatricians teamed up and presented the study of the RIT at the national conference of the Paediatrics Association of Nigeria the following January, 2004, in the city of Zaria. The news of the RIT was widely welcomed by the neonatologists at the conference. Many paediatricians had private discussions to network with me for possible future application of the technique at their various tertiary hospitals. One of the enthusiastic neonatologists was Dr Omog of Mubi Tertiary Hospital (MTH). I wished I could begin the gradual upgrade of all the systems I had previously reprogrammed at some of the tertiary hospitals, converting them to be powered with the newly invented RIT, at discounted costs to the willing hospitals. This information was made available to the hospitals and quite a few implemented the option.

RIT to the rescue

In November 2003, a tertiary hospital in Lantang had a management crisis emanating from a total breakdown of the SCBU due to lack of functional incubators. Radical young paediatricians were no longer prepared to continue to practise without proper incubator intervention in a unit where neonatal thermal stability must be maintained. The unit was led by a young consultant, Dr Lawal, who belonged to a new breed of revolutionary Nigerian professionals. Lawal understood that it was foolhardy to do neonatology with a 'hardware hot water bottle' in an era of digital incubators. He would not serve in an SCBU without functional incubators, and often complained: 'our babies are dying in their numbers with no solution in view, yet we deceive ourselves that we are doing neonatology'. Dr

Lawal had several outbursts, declaring: 'I am tired of endless sounds of wailing from our nursing mothers' room due to the constant news of the loss of their babies. The CMD should fix this problem or we close down this SCBU'.

The Head of the Department of Paediatrics and the rest of the faculty members of the Paediatrics Department sympathised with Dr Lawal. Jointly, they tabled an official complaint to Dr Danladi, the Chief Medical Director, asking him to provide immediate intervention without further delay. The CMD spoke sympathetically to the departmental team that presented the request, but had some genuine concerns: 'The Management of the hospital is aware of the problem at the SCBU, and as you may confirm, we have been providing money for the Works and Maintenance Unit to repair these incubators,' he said.

'But sir, how many of the ten failed incubators have these Maintenance/Works Department people been able to put back to work?' said Lawal. 'Do they report back to you at all? I can tell you, sir, these guys are so incompetent that it does not bother them that the death rate of neonates presenting at our SCBU has continued to rise. We need to replace these incubators with new ones.' Dr Danladi was a forthright gentleman. He could happily do as Dr Lawal requested, but could not figure out if Lawal was aware of the huge costs involved in purchasing an incubator, let alone ten of them.

'These systems cost a lot and honestly we have no budgetary allocation of funds to acquire new ones,' he said. 'Nevertheless, we will make some enquiries to see if we can find some money to buy one or two.'

Lawal was sad as they left the CMD's office. 'How could he be talking of buying only one incubator?' he said to his colleagues. 'What use would one incubator be in a SCBU which often has 25 neonates, mostly premature, along with an admission? If they cannot buy us enough incubators, it would be more honourable to discharge the patients and close the unit. This will enable people to know that we cannot care for premature babies, so they will stop bringing them to us.'

Lawal had a strong Christian belief that part of his duty was to do everything humanly possible to fight the cause of neonatal survival. He was determined to embarrass the hospital management.

After a few weeks of waiting, still with no new incubators, Lawal took a radical approach, taking the law into his own hands. He locked up the incubator bay of the SCBU and turned away all the patients. The hospital management team was embarrassed. The outrage caused by this quickly reached the presidency in Abuja, the Nigerian capital. The hospital received a call that the presidency had been informed of the crisis that was brewing. No CMD would want to be on the radar of the Federal Government, as this position was a presidential appointment. The hospital had had an earlier crisis that had embarrassed the government, threatening Danladi's job, so he might not survive this time if a decisive solution was not quickly found to settle the problem and calm the tensed atmosphere caused by weeping mothers. There were no other viable hospitals to handle such a specialised aspect of medical practice in the entire state of Plateau. One might wonder why government officials would put Dr Danladi under such pressure when they hadn't provided money for such expenditure.

Danladi phoned up Mr Francis, a medical equipment supplier in Southampton, United Kingdom. He had known him for some years. 'Mr Francis, I have urgent need to fix ten broken-down incubators in my hospital at Lantang, can you help, please?' Danladi inquired.

'Please fax me the make, brand and serial numbers of all the ten incubators so I can investigate the possibility of repairs,' Francis replied. This was done without delay, but Francis's next advice was a heavy blow to Danladi. He said, 'Based on the models and serial numbers you sent, I can reliably tell you that these machines are outdated and can never be renovated. I am afraid your best option would be to dump these systems and buy replacements'.

Danladi was shattered. He tried to get further clarification from Francis. The next comment from Francis was probably meant to be a joke, but it was devastating to Danladi. He said, 'You know what, my good friend you cannot be talking of such outdated systems as Isolette models C86 and C100. I will tell you what to do. Find a free space behind your hospital, dig a ditch and dump these systems there, as they are no longer useful or serviceable. I have brand new incubators that I can supply to you as soon as you can send the payment through'.

Danladi's hospital management had no immediate money to buy several incubators, so he was prepared for any solution. Dr Lawal had heard about the launch of the new RIT system at CCTH Enugu. He contacted the paediatricians at CCTH to explain the new repair technique that had been tested at their SCBU centre. He was happy with all that was said about the RIT system. 'I will tell my CMD about this good news, perhaps this will be an option for us,' he said.

Dr Lawal got my contact number and reached out to me. 'Can you come to see our CMD as we are in a serious crisis at the moment due to lack of functional incubators, please?' Dr Lawal asked. It was late October 2003.

Dr Danladi was pleasantly surprised to hear that I promised I could apply my new RIT technique to restore the ten incubators in 10 days. The cost for all ten incubators was only a fraction of the cost of two new ones as quoted by Mr Francis. Danladi did not hesitate. Francis had said these systems were no longer useful, so he had nothing to lose, even if they failed. However, if it worked, he would be a hero. So he took the extraordinary decision to convert the entire fleet of 10 malfunctioning incubators into RIT systems.

The contract was awarded and work commenced. This was the first application of the RIT on an industrial scale, testing the technology to its limit. Danladi could lose his job if things went wrong. He could bear this though, as he was already under investigation due to the poor state of the SCBU.

In fact the RIT successes at the Lantang Tertiary Hospital would later guarantee Danladi's job and prevent a premature termination of his appointment. This was a boost to the new technology and it opened up the era of having up to ten functional incubators at the same time in any Nigerian SCBU. Danladi was so pleased that he decided to sign a maintenance agreement with Pokaiz Engineering Limited and retain me as a visiting consultant. The Lantang success led to a number of other hospitals adopting the RIT and recovering many abandoned carcasses of old incubators.

Prior to the RIT era (in 2003), it was very rare to come across any Nigerian tertiary hospital with as many as five functional incubators at the same time. There could be up to

30 broken-down incubators in a hospital, scattered around the workshops, walkways and stores.

Whatever I could do for the Nigerian neonates with my RIT technique, it could only happen within the short periods of time I managed to take breaks from my studies to fly in from London. It was difficult, but I never relented.

How did RIT incubators compare with the modern incubators being marketed in Nigeria in terms of efficiency, longevity, ease of operation, maintainability and so on? This was a crucial question, which if properly answered would create an appropriate perspective on marketing for the RIT initiative. There was the need for a well-crafted research methodology for a comparative investigation of its performance against the other brands of modern incubators being used across some of the SCBUs within my Nigerian practice.

My research experience so far at the Royal was enough for me to design and initiate this study in collaboration with Dr Lawal and a few other Nigerian SCBU clinical friends at Enugu and Jalingo. The RIT had opened up a new enthusiasm for clinical collaboration in my work. My services were now in more demand from SCBUs across the country. The new opportunities opened up more jobs and increased my income. It looked like God was making special provision for me to keep up with my PhD costs and living maintenance in London.

The great disappointment

The consultancy fees I received from the Nigerian hospitals were my only source of income; they paid for my tuition and marginally supported my family. But the money was often insufficient. Iphii and I shed all the luxury and comfort we were accustomed to back home in Nigeria. We lived among the 'rich', but in students' apartments located around expensive areas of England such as South Kensington (SW7), Teddington (TW11) and Primrose Hill (NW1); however, we barely managed to put food on the table for our small family of three.

I held on for the successful completion of my MPhil transfer assessment, but without any financial support from my supervisors as promised. Every PhD research project at the Royal had to pass this transfer hurdle, normally within the first 15 months, before candidates could be given approval to continue to degree completion. Candidates must show that significant progress had been made towards answering the research question. They must also provide a convincing roadmap on how they could proceed to finish. A success at transfer assessment qualified the candidate for the degree of Master of Philosophy (MPhil). Successful candidates without funding could choose to drop out at this stage with a compensatory degree award of MPhil.

My team of assessors, led by Professor Duncan, were pleased with the amount of work that had been done. Duncan was particularly impressed that within the 15 months of the programme, I had already established a set of convincing fundamental computer codes that could guarantee a successful research investigation into the functions of the glenohumeral ligaments. The amiable Professor McDaniel was amazed at my progress, and agreed with the comments of the chief assessor, saying: 'It was a wonderful presentation, there is no doubt that Hippolite is capable of completing the PhD. It was quite impressive'. The assessors submitted their report to Royal

University, recommending that the transfer was a success; hence I could progress to the PhD finish line.

I relished every moment my success brought and became more hopeful that my supervisors would be happy to use their huge resources to source grants quickly, to enable me to refund the costs of the completed 15 months of study. Harry and Ricky were also excited, as they were both congratulated for my transfer success. It was a big relief that their student had passed this great hurdle at the Royal. The good news of the successful transfer assessment was received with joy by every person who was close to me, especially Iphii who had sacrificed a lot coping with my new busy lifestyle.

However, the excitement did not last long. Two weeks later, I was invited to my main supervisor's office for a meeting to discuss my funding and the future of my research. With a smile on my face as ever, I greeted my supervisors and took a seat. Harry chaired the meeting, sharing the excitement of the vast amount of my achievements within a short period of time, but regretted their inability to secure any grants up to the end of the transfer stage.

'I am not sure this programme can continue as we can no longer guarantee our ability to secure any funds for you, either now or in the foreseeable future,' said Harry. 'The Department is only too happy to award you the MPhil degree certificate for the work done so far.'

Harry and Ricky might have been sincere in persuading me to start a PhD programme with promises of funding. Nevertheless, I was heartbroken. My heart sank as though in sudden bereavement. I felt in my penury that I had wasted my money and time, and had been duped and betrayed by my Royal University confidants. How would I tell the story of dropping out of my PhD ambition to the numerous people back home who had felt I was crazy to embark on such a journey without securing the necessary funding? Would it not be more amusing to tell everyone that God had approved this programme? Several thoughts passed through my mind in a short time. I was deeply shaken. My faith was being put to a difficult test yet again by this development. There was dead silence, with everyone burying their faces in their hands.

'I am so sorry, Hippolite,' said Harry as Ricky looked on sadly. The tension in my head reverberated with a sudden headache. 'I am so sorry,' said Harry again. Still with my face buried in my hands, I remained speechless for a while. I could not cry, but my eyes had turned red under the stress. 'I really am so sorry for this,' said Harry again and again.

Finally I lifted my head to look at Harry and then Ricky: 'Okay,' I said in a quiet tone.

'What do you want to do now?' Harry asked. 'We can start the paperwork for the Royal MPhil certificate to be issued and officially terminate the PhD course, or do you want some time to think about any other steps?'

I had been wondering what my response would be in the unlikely event of this kind of worst-case scenario. Suddenly all the memories of the disappointing Nigerian events of 2000 and God's responses of 2001 came flooding my mind, motivating me to deliver a thrilling analogy of my situation. Still staring at Harry, I said: 'I have an idea and must cautiously apply wisdom. Do you still wish to supervise my PhD to completion, Harry?'

'Yes of course, except for this problem,' replied Harry.

My eyes red and soaked in tears, I said, 'I feel like the most unfortunate man on earth at the moment, but I will tell you how I picture myself in this whole ugly drama. I am like a poor dreamer on one bank of a mighty river who can barely swim but wants to cross to the opposite bank. Being handicapped by his inability to swim, he is considered to be over-ambitious and is ridiculed by his friends. Nevertheless the poor dreamer does not want to give up the idea, because his crossing would be of benefit to certain poor people who depend on the outcome of this mission. There is only one way of crossing the river, a little three-seater canoe piloted by two strangers he met on the riverbank. The two men persuade the Poor Dreamer to come on board and be helped. Unknown to the Dreamer, these two expert swimmer friends have conspired against him. They set off, but in the middle of the river, they intentionally capsize the vessel. They dive in and swim off. The Poor Dreamer, who cannot swim, initially sinks, but suddenly he is thrown up. Eyes and mouth open, he flails the water, expecting to drown. Meanwhile his other friends, who had tried to dissuade from crossing, have no pity for him. They taunt him and make fun of him even as his survival hangs by a thread.'

'The Dreamer knows there is no more help and he may drown, whether he swims on towards the other side or back to where he started. He must quickly apply wisdom to take a decision. If he struggles on the way back but escapes drowning, he will live the rest of his life with a sense of failure and be a laughing stock to his friends; on the other hand, if he moves on, he may die, but if not he will at least live to value his determination to make such a life-threatening sacrifice. He will end up a hero, proving his friends wrong, but above this, he will have achieved hope for the poor people who depend on his mission. If he drowns, many might still remember him as one who died fighting a just cause. Therefore, the Dreamer considered that the consequences of going back are worse than of going forward, so he decides to move forward in faith.'

Everyone remained quiet. My eyes were now dry but still very red. 'It is really sad that I have been so cruelly treated, Harry,' I continued. 'I do not know how this could be done, but I most certainly don't want your MPhil certificate. I already have two Masters' certificates in my CV, so what do I need your MPhil for? I don't need it as I will move on to complete my PhD. However, if I crash out at any point down the line I will be more proud of myself than if I pack my bags and quit at this stage'. With these words, I stood up and stormed out of Harry's office and headed for home.

The depression and mourning did not last for too long as I often reminded myself of my year 2000 disastrous decision to cancel my UK trip after the accident at Njaba Bridge. I quickly settled with what the reality held for me in my mind: 'I am engaged in a battle that is obviously overwhelming to me – I need God again to do what no man wants to do for me,' I prayed. 'For the sake of the Nigerian neonates I won't give up. My past, present and future is to strengthen their survival rates through efficient incubator application; any other activities, PhD inclusive, I consider secondary to this.' I would now strengthen my quarterly medical mission trips to Nigeria to serve the SCBUs that retained my services. I trusted that God would make hospital managements not hesitate or delay to settle my bills as these remained my only income for my PhD research and family maintenance. The future of my neonatal research ambitions for better understanding of peculiar neonatal militating factors in Nigeria must also be secured. Therefore I must devise a method of immediate deployment of all the research skills I was learning to investigate neonatal situations that could enable me understand neonatal physiology and thermoneutrality beyond mere incubator repairs. Securing the endorsement of certain Nigerian key clinical friends, I designed the methodology for the validation study of the 'recycled incubator technology (RIT)' and the other peer-reviewed studies that would follow.

God remained true for me as I studied full-time, paid my fees and looked after my family of three without any financial help from elsewhere. This was painstakingly achieved by a well-coordinated sandwiching of a regular period of travelling to Nigeria to execute my system maintenance contracts with a few hospitals. It was hard and burdensome but there was no other alternative for raising all the funds required in the UK, and at the same time contributing to my primary passion of neonatal survival in Nigeria. It was for the great grace of God that my activities remained relevant within the Nigerian practice even when I lived far away in the United Kingdom. The grace of God made it possible for the hospitals to pay me for my labours – no matter how long it took some stubborn CMDs to do this. Until now it had remained a great testimony of God's awesomeness, an amazing display of the fantastic God – that I attended Royal University London for nearly six years being completely self-supported. God did it for me! God did it for the Nigerian neonates! I studied under the best professors Royal University could afford at the time, acquiring superior training that would soon enhance my ability to carry out rigorous scientific investigations for the Nigerian neonate. My well-structured periods and time allotments for consulting in each of the few Nigerian hospitals that cared to employ my services became well-established. I could adequately identify neonatal research questions, investigating these and as well as managing other needs that presented as I improved on my skills at research.

Harry and Ricky loved my efficiency with the various segments of my research investigations. I understood what I wanted to achieve with my orthopaedic research and regularly reminded my supervisors that I had no room for failure. I would often insist on certain aspects of the research investigation I got attracted to. Sometimes my supervisors would view these as irrelevant but I insisted and followed my instincts, or perhaps God's guidance. I had my own future in focus, so I would not budge to any pressure from Harry or Ricky. However I tried to peacefully resolve my desires on every segment of the research topic provided these were within the content of the grand research question. I had a personal drive, and remained ambitious at work. I often rubbed in the fact that I was self-funded by saying: 'I pay the bills, so I should be allowed to take the decisions, especially if these contain no damaging sides against my research'. I studied a number of semi-independent aspects of the anatomy and biomechanics of the shoulder joint. Each of these independent investigations were fantastically stand-alone publishable pieces of scientific information that eventually came together to make the extra-ordinary volume of my PhD.

After successful completion of the PhD research in 2006

– a work that independently rolled out 11 separate scientific journal papers – I was reemployed as a post-doctoral researcher at the Orthopaedic Biomechanics Section of Royal University London. During the succeeding years, the Bioengineering Department, the Institute of Biomedical Engineering and the Department of Surgery and Cancer re-employed me at various times as a research associate, a crossover consultant orthopaedics biomechanist or a research fellow. The conditions for my employment in each of these research positions were structured to respect my well-known passion for the Nigerian neonatal work. Hence, the research positions I occupied were designed not to interfere with the Nigerian consultancy.

CHAPTER 7

BETWEEN THE LECTURE THEATRE AND THE FRONT LINE

✦✦✦✦✦✦✦

Iremained a research staff member of the Bioengineering Department of Royal University for many years; however, I often had to review my association whenever the opportunity called in order to remain focused on my neonatal vision whilst retaining my relevance at Royal. My Nigeria consultancy among the tertiary hospitals required proper redefinition to differentiate me from other contractors that hung around the hospitals, seeking all kinds of jobs. My collaborations with the Nigerian paediatricians were becoming more clinical as well than the basic technical supports I provided them. We jointly began to investigate strange phenomena perceived to have direct or indirect effects on the survival of neonates. It became more fitting to address me with the title of 'visiting consultant' as I continued to spread my operational reach to many other tertiary hospitals across the entire landscape of Nigeria.

Harry remained my most influential post-PhD mentor as I translated all my Royal University orthopaedics research skills into new frontiers for African neonatal research. It was not an easy challenge, but I had acquired a lot of experience in independent research under the tutelage of the great Professor Harry. I boldly questioned observed phenomena at the Nigerian SCBUs, and designed and initiated research investigations to understand these. Local paediatricians and chief medical directors across the hospitals gladly collaborated, and co-authored a number of these findings in reputable scientific journals. Professor Sotus's earlier advice as I contemplated dropping my Royal PhD subject was thus validated: indeed I had been trained through orthopaedics research by Professor Harry, but I was aiming at becoming a champion in neonatology research. I particularly designed studies that were aimed at investigating factors that related to temperature stability and control in the newborn.

My research team of willing Nigerian paediatricians and neonatologists was now growing in numerical strength. The two levels (I and II) of my developed training courses for neonatal nurses and doctors had been well-established in some hospitals and were being executed effectively. Every year, streams of cohorts were recruited into the courses at the various tertiary hospitals. Certificates were awarded to successful candidates after end-of-course examinations conducted locally at each hospital. A number of completed collaborative research studies were also being peer-reviewed and published in respected international journals. It might have been unfortunate that Harry and Ricky failed to obtain a study grant for me, but I felt my present African neonatal research – considered excellent by many reviewers – would not have materialised if it had not been for Harry's great academic qualities, which had rubbed off on me. Harry was a great academic who knew how to be excited by every discovery or piece of progress. I will often say of my supervisor: 'Harry was funny and a delight. I so well mastered his emotional threats that I manipulated this to my advantage during my PhD studentship. If I wanted Harry's immediate attention, I would simply call him and say, 'Harry, I've got some good news'. Notice of new insight into a research question could easily turn Harry on. He would immediately think I had discovered something new in my research and would never hesitate to ask me to come over to his office at the earliest opportunity. Sometimes he would storm into my own office to soak up whatever excitement the moment held. Harry really taught me how to celebrate discoveries! There was another excellent side to this great man's attitude towards the celebration of new discoveries – it never lasted too long! His attitude was to celebrate and quickly 'piggy-bank' this and then chase up the next target. I was already a hard worker before my arrival at the Royal, but Harry taught me to 'horse-work'. I will eternally remain thankful to Harry. He might not be aware of it, but his tough personality helped to bring out the best of my scholastic quality and passion for the African neonate.'

After many years on the Royal orthopaedics biomechanics research staff – most of the time within Harry's group – I was still unable to accept a switch-over to the teaching staff status, as such a position would undermine my Nigerian work. Harry felt this was a huge sacrifice because my progress as a university academic was being compromised, he feared. The Royal, as a global top university, did not allow 'absentee' lecturers, as was often the case among Nigerian universities. The life of every Royal lecturer revolved around the student calendar; hence, it was impossible for me to take up a teaching role at Royal due to my frequent trips to Nigeria.

One day, Professor Harry invited me for a discussion. 'Hippolite,' he said, 'Your frequent absence from the UK has remained a difficult barrier to your progress as an academic biomechanist in this department. I am worried about this and I am beginning to think that your future in the Royal might well lie within paediatric practice; we may have to find a way of progressing your career in this department along this course'.

Initially, I felt looked down on for this implication that I was no longer fit for orthopaedics. However as I thought about Harry's words I was convinced he was right. Hence, I welcomed the proposal and encouraged Harry to go ahead with whatever plans he was contemplating. Later that year Professor Harry became the Head of the Department of Bioengineering and went ahead to establish a virtual 'Centre for Frugal Medical Technology for low- and middle-income countries'. This was created to enable a new research position for me to be set up, to officially convert my African neonatal research exploits into Royal University academic points. My new title became 'Honorary Research Fellow'. This was a very senior position, but there were no teaching responsibilities attached. Professor Harry hoped that the newly-established Centre would develop into a unique capacity-building model in medical technology for Africa – along the direction in which my research was evolving. The model targeted indigenous young African people who were resident in their African countries for studentship at the Royal. Candidates would be admitted for postgraduate coursework in the Bioengineering Department in London, but their complementary degree projects would be carried out in their own African countries – projects that would apply local content whilst addressing local African medical problems. I was to ensure that the initial efforts of the African scheme were channelled towards neonatal projects. The Royal Centre considered this initiative to be what a true African technological empowerment should be. Professor Harry was committed to ensuring this happened.

RIT help for the neonates

As many as 12 tertiary hospitals in Nigeria applied my old incubator reprogramming technique between 1996 and 2003. This was an era when it was a big achievement for a SCBU to demonstrate the availability of as many as five functional incubators. The reprogramming technique made it possible for just a few to maintain a fleet of five incubators or more; these were the tertiary hospitals at Enugu, Calabar, Port Harcourt, Aba, Jos and Sokoto. Though few, these incubators made a great difference to their neonatal outcomes as compared to having no functional systems at all. The few hospitals that retained my visiting consultancy position were proud to be able to keep this number consistently functional.

It was not possible for me to provide retained services at all the hospitals due to frequent disagreements with powerful individuals at some centres which made this difficult. I could not waste the little time I had during the years of my full-time studies at Royal University engaging in battles with these people, so I concentrated my services at the hospitals where the CMDs were truly passionate about saving the neonates. Notable among these was Professor Etawo of Igweocha. The incubators at many other centres where I had stopped going were starting to break down again due to poor maintenance, so many SCBUs were losing the ground they had gained earlier when I had been resident in Nigeria.

I was not necessarily keen on maintaining systems that had been powered by my old reprogramming technique after the launch of the RIT. However, the application of the new technique among the numerous Nigerian tertiary hospitals was going at a very slow pace and only three hospitals had applied the newly-invented RIT system by 2005. This was not encouraging, and I used every opportunity to try to persuade hospitals to upgrade their systems.

One such opportunity came six months after the successful clinical trial of the RIT at Enugu Tertiary Hospital. It was at the 2004 annual scientific conference of the Paediatrics Association of Nigeria in the northern Nigeria city of Zaria. I was invited to deliver a talk on 'digitally upgraded incubators – an economic alternative to modern systems in Africa'. Among those in the audience was Dr Omogbenga (Omog), the chairman of Medical Advisory Committee of the Mubi Tertiary Hospital (MUTH). Through his position, Omog was deputy to the Chief Medical Director. His title was popularly referred to as 'CMAC'. He was also the consultant in charge of the special care baby unit. He was a kind and God-fearing gentleman.

My talk at the Zaria conference was evidence based. The claims in my paper presentation were right on the spot, confirmed by a number of attendees from the hospitals cited in the paper. These were very senior colleagues such as Professor Ozubu from Enugu and Professor Mabok from Port Harcourt. It was a great image boost for me at national level. Dr Omog and many other participants could not wait for the session to end, as they wanted to have one-on-one discussions with me, all presenting the overwhelming burden of the lack of functional incubators. Omog approached me to ask if I could consider coming to the rescue of the Mubi neonatal unit. I agreed and scheduled a visit to the hospital during my fourth quarter consulting trip in October 2004.

Omog returned to Mubi with the exciting news and agreed on the implementation of this project with the Chief Medical Director, Dr Kature. It had always been an embarrassment for Dr Kature that his SCBU never had a functional incubator despite the status of the hospital as an institution for training would-be consultant neonatologists. It baffled Kature that his predecessors could complete their entire tenures in office and leave the SCBU as they found it, without functional incubators. He had been under consistent pressure to improve this situation since Dr Omog became his CMAC.

Kature promised Omog that it would be his pleasure to improve the ugly situation of not having functional incubators, but the machines were very expensive and not affordable within the meagre funds allocations from the government. Kature managed to purchase one incubator before the conference where Omog met me. Dr Omog however was aware that one incubator for an SCBU of up to 25-cot capacity was little more than a joke. 'One new incubator is better than nothing, and also a step in the positive direction,' he would encourage himself. He wondered how much longer it would be before the hospital could muster some millions of naira to purchase one more incubator.

The great testimonies of the RIT at the Zaria Paediatrics conference sounded like the kind of miracle Omog had been hoping for to transform his practice at the Mubi SCBU. The money-saving technique that could help in restoring dead incubators and making them functionally new for less than 20% of the cost of new ones was the perfect option.

'Did the conference go well?' asked Dr Kature as Dr Omog stepped into his office to greet him after returning from the conference.

'It was fantastic, especially because I met someone whose presentation was a pleasant surprise to many paediatricians – a UK-based biological engineer who could transform dead incubators into new ones at very low cost,' he reported with a beaming smile.

Kature was rather surprised when Omog told him how many respectable neonatologists had applied the RIT and my previous reprogramming technologies – including the renowned Professor Azubuike of the National Postgraduate Medical College of Nigeria – and how they attested to the efficiency and reliability of the systems.

'Don't you think we need him here?' Kature asked Omog. 'Were you able to invite him? I guess many of your colleagues must have rushed to entice him to their own hospitals.' Kature knew that he was not alone in having the problem of poor neonatal incubator facilities. He was actually the chairman of a special national club of the CMDs of Federal Government-owned tertiary hospitals. The CMDs' club was a well-organised association that became more powerful while Kature was their chairman. Members regularly met to exchange ideas and encourage one another as they faced the challenges of the difficult job of being the chief executive of a tertiary hospital in Nigeria. Kature knew that inadequacy of functional incubators was a nightmare shared by most of his colleagues in the club.

An eighth wonder of the world

Kature signed an official invitation inviting my company to recycle four old incubators at the Mubi SCBU. He looked forward to a positive outcome from my visit as this would also be of benefit to his many colleagues in the CMDs' club. Beyond the Mubi need he needed to try me first before tabling this at his CMDs' club. The chairmanship of the club left him with the responsibility of coordinating meetings where his members discussed any identified successful solutions at national level. Kature thought it sounded like a solution to be promoted at national level if it worked at his Mubi SCBU.

A few months later, before I began the incubator project implementation, the CMD of Benin City Tertiary Hospital, Professor Gregory, visited the Mubi hospital during a short faculty accreditation assignment. Gregory was sorry to notice that the hospital had no functional incubators in the wards, yet the shells of obsolete ones could be seen lying all around. This was the kind of sight he was quite used to, except that these were almost being used as dustbins instead of being put away neatly in stores or workshops. He was not too surprised, since his own hospital at Benin was in a similar situation.

Dr Kature began to tell Professor Gregory that he had confirmed that the Lantang hospital, headed by Dr Danladi, had a fleet of up to 10 functional incubators through the work of a UK-based Nigerian doctor. Just like Kature, Gregory was a passionate and honest professional who would do anything within his ability to help in lowering neonatal mortality at his hospital. As they walked along the hospital corridors, passing by the abandoned old incubators, Kature said, 'These carcasses that are lying all over the place will soon be restored as fully functional incubators in a few months from now, when the UK doctor comes around'.

His enthusiasm as he spoke of repairing the incubators was rather amusing to Gregory, especially when he saw that some of the machines Kature was referring to had all kinds of junk inside them. 'I beg your pardon,' said Gregory. 'Are you referring to these dustbins or some other systems?'

'Yes of course, these incubators,' replied Kature.

'Do you call these incubators? It will be the eighth wonder of the world for these to ever nurse a baby again. Please notify me about this if it ever happens,' Gregory said.

'I certainly will,' promised Kature.

In October 2004, I arrived to begin work on the four carcasses that had been assembled. The project was completed within a week of arrival, and all four incubator carcasses were restored to glory as RIT systems, all for less than the cost of one new incubator. It was celebration time for Dr Omog and Dr Kature.

'This will be one of the smartest money-saving decisions

we have ever made during my tenure as CMAC,' Omog said to me.

'I am glad, and it has been my great pleasure to be of help, my dear sir,' I replied in my posh half-British accent.

I could be seen soaking up the happy atmosphere as people gave me handshakes for a job well done. Kature was probably the most visibly excited person as this was like scoring a point where his predecessors in office had all failed. He could now boast of having functional incubators in his SCBU – not just one or two but a total of five.

Kature was so happy for me, 'Thank you, thank you,' he said over and over again. 'Ahhh I remember,' he added, pointing his finger in the air, 'I will call Gregory, my Benin friend, to give him some news he might not be expecting. One of my CMD colleagues from Benin, an obs & gynae professor, said it would be the eighth wonder of the world for these pieces of junks to ever work again, so he must come and see this'. This remained a time of excitement for Dr Omog and Dr Kature, who did not waste time in calling Professor Gregory to break the news of his 'eighth wonder of the world'.

In November 2005, a couple of months after the Mubi job, my mobile phone rang repeatedly, displaying an unknown Nigerian number. It was Professor Gregory.

'I got your number from the Tertiary Hospital of Mubi, from my friend Doctor Kature,' he said. I have heard of the great job you did for them and wonder if you could schedule my own hospital, as we have similar needs at Benin City Tertiary Hospital.' I did not hesitate to scheduling the BCTH because things seemed to move faster with these Nigerian hospitals when the CMD, on his own, initiated the move following a situation of dire need. There were only five incubators in Kature's fleet because his hospital did not accumulate or retain too many carcases of previously failed incubators. They were disposing the systems off as scrap, and I found only four there. This was not so with Gregory's Benin hospital, where many years of replacing failed incubators after several repair attempts had left the hospital with a large fleet of obsolete and malfunctioning systems.

I was conducted around the various places where these could be found. There were about 13 of them, in the maintenance workshop, the hospital scrapyard, the store room of the paediatrics department and along walkways. However, I could find only one functional incubator running in the entire SCBU ward, one which had been newly purchased and had been in use at the Unit for about four months.

Gregory was happy to welcome me to his hospital. He explained what a nightmare it had been managing a big teaching hospital with only one functional incubator.

'Some of my CMD colleagues might decide to ignore this need, but, as you may be aware, by my medical speciality as a professor of obstetrics, it is difficult for me when I see the mothers going home without living babies,' he said. 'If you are able to repeat what I have hear you have done elsewhere, then I stand a chance of having as many functional incubators as we have carcases littered all over our premises.'

I loved Gregory's positive attitude, and I promised to assist in recycling as many machines as the hospital was willing to put back to work. The recycling project was carried out in batches of two or three incubators at a time, allowing a period of up to six months between each. Gregory was so committed to the project that he was able to achieve an incubator capacity of six systems by the end of 2006. By 2008 this had grown to eleven and it became the second SCBU with more than ten functional incubators at that time in Nigeria – the first being Tertiary Hospital Port Harcourt, where Professor Uriah had earlier collaborated with me to achieve a fleet of 13 functional incubators.

Gregory was very proud of achieving this within a year of getting to know me. Both Gregory and Kature were delighted with the performance of the RIT technology so far. However, the two agreed that a little more time was needed to confirm its performance longevity at their various centres. They agreed with me that provision of adequate functional incubators was a fundamental factor in tackling the fight against the high neonatal mortality rate in Nigeria. Gregory often expressed negative feelings about Millennium Development Goal target No.4 owing to the neonatal component. He would often say that there would be bad news about MDG(4) by 2015 if the high neonatal mortality problem was not solved quickly.

Doctor Kature, congratulating me for the successful two years of RIT service at his SCBU in 2007, said to me, 'This will definitely restore our confidence in effectively pushing performance boundaries for the MDG4 vision.'

Kature was delighted, as the Chairman of the CMDs' club, to invite me to deliver a presentation on the RIT systems at the general conference of the club in July 2007, hosted by Professor Gregory at Benin. The meeting was well attended by many chief executives of tertiary hospitals across Nigeria. Members of the CMDs' club were so impressed with the testimonies of members who were already applying the RIT in their various hospitals. Following the presentation, I was highly praised for my great contribution towards Nigeria's national development. The club finally passed a resolution to official adopt the RIT for use in member hospitals to fight high neonatal mortality. Members of the CMDs' club were encouraged to individually identify themselves to me to ensure that their respective hospitals benefited from the established corporate collaboration of the club with Pokaiz Engineering Limited.

Also present at this meeting was Dr Bellowa, the CMD of Nguru Tertiary Hospital. Dr Bellowa was delighted to hear all the testimonies concerning the RIT systems; however, he regretted that Professor Akiola was absent from the meeting. Akiola was the CMD of Ekiti Tertiary Hospital (ETHF) in Funtua, who had previously mentioned this new technique to Dr Bellowa during a telephone conversation.

CHAPTER 8

THE NEONATE 'WARRIORS'

✦✦✦✦✦✦✦

In December 2006, more than six months before the CMD club resolution of July 2007 in Benin city, Professor Akiola was still in his first 100 days in office as the new CMD of the Ekiti Tertiary Hospital, Funtua. He had inherited a number of troubled departments and units from the previous management of the hospital, and was still coming to terms with the reality of not having a single functional incubator in the entire hospital. He had previous experience as a businessman and had a business degree in addition to his medical degrees. Akiola considered his skills in medical economics would enable his success in office. He made a number of enquiries about neonatal devices, including a call to Dr Omog of Mubi Tertiary

Hospital concerning me. In his response to Akiola's enquiries, Omog said: 'Yes I know Hippolite very well. He came here to our hospital and astonished everyone. The old abandoned carcasses of incubators that no one considered would ever be useful again are all like brand new incubators now, thanks to Dr Hippolite. We have been using them for nearly two years, and I can tell you we all love the performance of the systems – they are magical. Dr Hippolite is fantastically skilfull and will never disappoint you if you wish to engage with him.'

After a couple of other calls with similar positive responses, Professor Akiola made up his mind to invite me and my Pokaiz Engineering team. He consulted some of the senior staff of his Works Department, excitedly telling them about me. Mr Jimo, the senior technician, did not look too pleased to hear my name.

'Jimo, you talked about how worried you had been about the lack of functioning incubators, yet you don't seem to be happy about the news of this great discovery I have made; do you know the man?' asked Professor Akiola.

'Yes sir, I know him, and I don't think he is as fantastic as you are presenting him. He has been here before, quarrelling with every person in our department,' replied Jimo. Jimo remembered how one of his colleagues, Mr Goke, had received a query in 2002 because of me. After consulting with his mates at the Works Department about his encounter with the new CMD over me, some did not quite remember who I was, although others, like Mr Goke, did.

'Remember that arrogant Mr Hippolite who doesn't like anyone to know what he does?' said Jimo. 'Whenever he receives his payment, he just takes his money and goes away without even a 'thank you' or the offer of an 'envelope' to appreciate us,' said Jimo. Mr Jimo and his colleagues saw me as a big threat, especially now I was being addressed as 'Doctor', so Jimo resolved to do everything to stop the CMD from inviting me to ETHF.

The CMD was surprised and disappointed that many of his staff in the Works department seemed to have this negative opinion about me while clinical fellows around Nigeria sang my praises. He felt that something must be wrong somewhere. For Akiola, personal differences between individuals must not stand in the way of restoring a functional SCBU at his hospital.

Akiola said to his CMAC as they discussed the strange reactions from Works Department: 'This must be an act of envy against this Dr Hippolite. I am not prepared to allow this to stand in my way in finding the solution for my broken-down incubators. I must not allow this SCBU to mess me up as it did my predecessors'.

Whilst Professor Akiola was making all these enquiries, the chairman of his hospital's Management Board, Emeritus Professor Umeagah, was independently asking around for possible solutions to the incubator problem. Professor Umeagah did not hesitate to contact me after Professor Norman of Asaba Tertiary Hospital spoke to him about me and my new RIT invention.

I went to Funtua during my next consulting trip to Nigeria at the invitation of Chairman Umeagah. Professor Akiola had also decided to contact me on the same issue, but he had no idea that his Board Chairman was a step ahead of him. Both men were later to argue who it was who actually brought Hippolite to ETHF, as one or the other was being praised for bringing the person who delivered the successes that ETHF achieved. It was, however, a great coincidence that both the Chairman of Board and the CMD had favoured the award of a contract to me for the restoration of some of the incubators.

This did not go down well with many 'caterpillars' who considered me an uncompromising and non-cooperative fellow, simply because I would never give bribes. They insisted on voting against any proposal to engage me. Most of the conspirators were technical staff whose inputs in such decisions were normally given serious consideration. Owing to this division of opinion, and the 'no' answers without very strong reasons, the CMD decided to disregard their negative recommendation. However, he would not risk the finances of the hospital to save himself from blame in case of failure. Hence, the CMD opted for awarding the contract to me but based on 'zero financial liability' to ETHF until seven months of successful usage of the recycled incubators had passed, followed by independent assessments of clinical outcomes and the continued functionality of the systems.

By this arrangement, I was not going to be financially enabled to execute the job. Worse still, I would not receive any payment for a minimum of seven months after the commissioning of the completed job. This amounted to borrowing a large sum of money to execute it. However, I was confident of the outcome of this challenge. I was determined to fight on for the neonates, even at the detriment of my finances.

Professor Akiola expected a negative response from me on his strange conditions, so he was thrilled when I agreed. The Ekiti Tertiary Hospital finally invited me officially when Akiola initiated what he referred to as 'the incubator project' in January 2007. It was more or less an executive order to get me involved, since for some unclear reason, perhaps based on tribal sentiments and my personality principles, some of Akiola's officers did not agree that this was the right decision to take.

During a follow-up meeting, Akiola re-emphasised to me: 'Based on my enquiries, I believe that you are capable of helping me to resolve this incubator issue, but I do not have the full support of my team'. The Professor reiterated the content of the contract narrative, emphasising: 'So, I am happy to start this project with you if you are still prepared to take all the initial financial risks, all by yourself. I will issue an approval so that ETHF will allow you to carry out the recycling of up to 10 incubators from the stock of 35 malfunctioning systems we have at various locations within the hospital. However, the hospital will not pay any money towards any stage of the project until the finished systems have been put to work for a minimum of six months. The final condition is a satisfactory report on full reassessment of the ten systems in terms of acceptability of performance by the Paediatrics Department after six months of usage.'

The large population of Funtua and the neighbouring states made ETHF a potential centre for the influx of needy neonates and hence crucial for the campaign to increase Nigerian neonate survival. Someone had to take a crucial risk for the survival of these poor babies, and I was happy to so do. Hence, in January 2007 I obtained a loan through my UK Virgin credit card and initiated the recycling of the incubators at ETHF. Professor Akiola gave his personal promise to be committed to this project all through his tenure in office if the initial test was successful. It was, and Akiola officially launched his 'incubator project initiative'. He would later go on to expand the incubator capacity of ETHF to become the largest unit amongst all Nigerian hospitals by far – a whopping 46 functional thermoneutral systems at the time of his hand over of ETHF management in October 2014.

Professor Akiola was a dignified personality with an impeccable passion for neonatal survival, and he religiously kept to his original promise without compromise.

Thus, a fleet of the first ten incubators were reintroduced into service at ETHF by the first week of February 2007.

More incubators for the ETHF

The success of the initial ten systems made ETHF Management strengthen its collaboration commitment. A very strong friendship between Akiola and me began to develop as we worked together to turn around the fortunes of the SCBU. My consultancy position at ETHF was formalised through my company. PEL was officially commissioned to utilize the hospital's large fleet of abandoned malfunctioning incubators to attempt to provide an adequate number of functional incubators in ETHF's three sections for neonatal nursing, i.e. Isi Ward, Aka Ward and Ukwu Ward. Ukwu Ward was the smallest of the three, being dedicated to the management of neonates undergoing treatment in the paediatric surgical section. Aka Ward, at a separate location, managed neonates referred from other hospitals. A mandatory six-monthly maintenance servicing of all recovered incubators was initiated and meticulously implemented all through the remaining seven and a half years of Akiola's tenure in office, at a fixed cost that was never upwardly reviewed all through the period. This failure-preventive audit culture (FAC) ensured the sustainability of acquired incubator capacity whilst more systems were being recycled and added to the fleet.

ETHF's 'incubator project initiative' also attracted external donations from other organizations that wished to identify with the achieved successes. This provided up to eight additional systems, making a total of 38 functional incubators at the ETHF's facilities. A total of eight units of neonatal resuscitaires were also acquired, making a grand total of 46 functional thermoneutral systems. The combined ETHF centres thus became the largest neonatal incubator capacity anywhere in Nigeria and, perhaps West Africa, as at July 2014.

My popularity at ETHF soared, and I attracted donations of other useful items of neonatal care at various times during the years of Akiola's tenure. These came from individuals and organizations that were impressed by my medical outreaches in Nigeria. These items included baby weighing scales, neonatal apnoea monitors, incubators and digital timers. Full elective training courses on paediatrics incubation technique were conducted at various times all through Professor Akiola's years, with an average of 25 participants per stream in attendance. The various streams of course cohorts came from the nursing, technical and clinical divides. The costs of the courses were always funded by the United Kingdom supporters of my work, which included Hornchurch Baptist Church of Essex, England, so the ETHF did not have to pay any money for all the staff that passed through the courses all through the years Akiola served as the CMD.

The successes of Akiola's incubator project initiative made a great impact on the ETHF SCBUs' confidence to handle challenging neonatal cases. This comprised, amongst others, an improved success rate for managing multiple births, including quintuplets. Mr Kelechi was the senior management staff that Akiola appointed to manage the administration of the incubator-project to ensure its unhindered success. Kelechi was selfless and served the full interests of the CMD and my principles, ensuring that the 'caterpillars' were kept away from frustrating the project. Kelechi was a true anchor for the neonates at this large facility.

Nobleman Bellowa of Yobe

'In a room of absolute darkness, it can often be challenging to accept that there could still be shiny objects lying around'. This is a common saying in Amuchaland, the birthplace of my father. At a time in Nigeria when chief executives of government establishments enriched themselves to the detriment of national development; when many resorted to violence and wanton destruction of lives and public properties through bombing and terrorising Boko Haram Islamic militants, a noble man, Doctor Bellowa, saw his new appointment as a rare opportunity to display a different spirit of hospital management performance in Nigeria.

Nguru was an abandoned ancient Nigerian city in Yobe State in north-east Nigeria. It used to be a popular colonial railway city for the transport of economic products to the southern seaports for export to colonial England. Up until 2014 the tertiary hospital at Nguru (NGTH) remained the most difficult-to-reach federal tertiary hospital in Nigeria. The roads were impassable and the terrorist activities of Boko Haram Islamic terrorists exacerbated the lack of interest of Nigerian professionals from the mainland cities in visiting NGTH Nguru, let alone taking up any available job opportunities therein, or to live in the town. Hence, the undesirable partners – some dishonest Federal Ministry of Health staff from Abuja – were less willing to go to NGTH Nguru as they visited other hospitals in their drives to twist the hands of hospital chief executives, pilfering funds. The bad roads and fear of terrorists made Nguru unattractive for the so-called 'monitoring visits' by federal staff for a long time. This could have given great freedom to any corrupt Chief Medical Director at NGTH to short-change the establishment and divert funds to personal pockets. On the other hand, the poor federal 'radar' could be an advantage for an honest CMD wishing to achieve big developments for the common people without fund depletion by visiting federal staff. An old colonial hospital site in Nguru had remained the site for this federal hospital for many years whilst funds meant for development were poorly managed year after year by successive CMDs. The hospital had no resident consultants for many years, despite the huge sums of federal allocation money given to the CMDs each year.

Doctor Bellowa was incorruptible, unassuming and kind-hearted. He became the CMD of NGTH in 2006 and decided to do things differently. Fifteen months into his first four-year tenure in office, he attended the CMD club conference in Benin City, where he listened to my presentation on the RIT systems. He was impressed, but felt reluctant to approach me. He reasoned that bad roads make it very difficult for people to come to Nguru, otherwise it would have been good to ask this British expert to come to help.

Dr Bellowa regretted the inaccessible roads. He wished there were no Boko Haram threats. He wished Nguru was a city with big hotels. All these were impediments, without which a great opportunity existed if this man could come to NGTH, his sorry thoughts continued. This elegant professional from London would surely not want to come as far as this poor, remote village. All the odds and doubts were crowding into Bellowa's mind. He could not approach me. He had inherited not a single functional incubator from his predecessors and his attempt to purchase two units had ended up in the hands of fraudulent marketers and yielded no results. He wished Nguru was developed enough with adequate hotels to host this sophisticated London expatriate in order to make it possible for this new incubator solution to be applied at NGTH. He assumed that the luxuries of hotel accommodation would be as important to me as my passion for the lives of these poor neonates. The threats posed by Boko Haram terrorists also seemed a serious impediment.

He could not approach me directly with any requests, but he pleaded with the chairman of the CMDs' club, Dr Kature, to speak to me about Nguru's needs. Bellowa had been determined to embark on revolutionary hospital development programmes as soon as he was appointed to the office of CMD at NGTH. He wanted to embark on the construction of a brand-new hospital complex to relocate the entire NGTH. Federally-funded projects to relocate various federal tertiary hospitals from temporary sites to permanent ones were happening all over the country. Some dishonest government officials, compelling or conniving with some CMDs, cunningly diverted fund allocations meant for actualising these projects, and many of the projects consumed billions of naira in money without completion, passing through successive CMDs in office. The NGTH was to be the only exception, because Bellowa had fundamentally initiated this project at Nguru and locally mobilised his in-house architects and builders, implementing the project to a successful completion, all within his first four-year term in office. He began the process of relocating the various hospital departments towards the end of this period.

I promised the chairman of the CMDs' club that I was prepared to go any length for the neonates, no matter where they might be, provided there was a willing CMD to make this happen. The location of Nguru would not be an impediment, I reassured the Chairman. Doctor Bellowa returned from the conference and shared the news of the RIT and the man behind it with his 'top management committee' (TMC) at NGTH. The hospital's deputy CMD, Dr Bawa, was an internet-loving young man. He loved his mobile phones and always played around with the latest internet-enabled phones, even in the remote village of Nguru. He could easily surf the internet for the latest news and verification of claims. The CMD's excitement and the manner of his description of 'Dr Hippolite and his RIT' raised curiosity among all TMC members present, including Dr Bawa, who thought that if these claims were true, the internet must have something to say about this fellow.

'What did you say this person's name is?' he asked.

'Hippolite, Doctor Hippolite Amadi,' replied the CMD. Dr Bawa typed the name into the Google search engine of his mini laptop computer. This returned several results in half a second.

He opened one of the listed links with a picture and turned around the screen of his computer towards the CMD.

'Is this the man you met in Benin City?' asked Dr Bawa.

'Absolutely, that is the man,' replied the CMD.

'Okay, I will read what the internet has to say about him.' Dr Bawa read a little from a Royal University London page. He suddenly stopped and looked up. 'Ladies and gentlemen, this man is a great researcher from a top and prestigious university. I doubt this top professional would want to come to our remote location here in Nguru, but if he agrees, we must take the opportunity.'

The CMD club's chairman telephoned Dr Bellowa and encouraged him to contact me if NGTH was still interested. A couple of weeks later, I received an invitation from the NGTH. I was happy to initiate Bellowa's incubator project in Nguru in March 2008 with the recycling of four available casings of old incubators. My incubator consultancy at NGTH lasted all through the remaining years of Bellowa's eight years in office.

Just like Professor Akiola, Dr Bellowa was passionate about the survival of the neonates and hence displayed extraordinary interest in any research that could provide more clues and better outcomes. Bellowa was a consultant obstetric surgeon, but his extraordinary passion for neonatal survival was far bigger than any interest I had seen in other paediatricians around Nigeria. Despite being the most remotely located and looked-down-upon federal tertiary hospital – without a single resident consultant paediatrician – NGTH participated with high quality contributions in many of my neonatal research investigations between 2009 and 2015. The SCBU had not existed before Bellowa's tenure. However, within a few years, the Nguru SCBU became an attraction for visitors coming to the new hospital facility, such that bigger and older northern Nigeria tertiary hospitals visited Nguru to copy developmental ideas, including the building plan of the SCBU. By the end of 2013 the SCBU of Nguru had grown to become the northern Nigerian centre with the largest fleet of functional neonatal incubators.

Bellowa's zeal for the neonates was so deep that I once asked him why he was more passionate than the paediatricians, whose direct patients these neonates were. The CMD replied, 'Doctor, you may understand that as an obstetrician/gynaecologist, I could have known these tiny patients more than seven months longer than the paediatricians. So in fact, they should be dearer to me than to the paediatricians, and I am bound to do everything possible for their survival. Moreover, I would not derive any greater joy from my work than to see my own patients – their mothers – return home with their babies alive'.

'That was an awesome answer,' I said. However, I never stopped wondering why many other 'obs & gynae' doctors I had met during my long career were not as compassionate towards this neonatal crisis as I had seen displayed in Bellowa's practice.

In 2011, Bellowa set up the HippoliteNGTH centre for neonatal research, spearheading the scientific investigation that identified how neonatal evening-fever syndrome (EFS) could be eradicated in Nigeria.

The NGTH Nguru adopted virtually all the mitigating procedures already developed through my research work to combat high neonatal mortality in Nigerian facilities. Hence, Dr Bellowa initiated the use of apnoea monitors to support all incubator-dependent neonates and other premature neonates being nursed in the incubators and cots. This helped in saving many of the neonates that tended to die from incessant apnoeic attacks. This practice was made to become the SCBU standard throughout the period Bellowa was the CMD. Nguru was the first Nigerian SCBU to simultaneously operate two sets of power banking system (PBS). This was power supply technology that ensured the continuous operation of the incubators and other thermoneutral systems in the SCBU during mains failures. Unannounced power cuts at Nigerian hospitals could often last more than ten hours at a stretch, shutting down life-support devices, including the incubators. Frequent power cuts contributed to the mortality of many neonates in Nigeria due to hypothermia that occurred when incubators suddenly stopped. Failed power supply frequently damaged neonatal systems such as the incubators and, as I discovered from my research, this became a major contributing factor to early neonatal deaths. I organised frequent training courses on incubator interventions and neonatal thermoneutral control, refreshing the knowledge of the clinical and nursing staff members of the SCBU and the entire paediatrics department. Bellowa also made certain doctors and nurses from the obs & gynae department attend these courses in order to understand the new procedures being operated at the SCBU. This fostered better functional links between the two sections of the hospital, especially in the manner of neonatal transfer from the labour ward theatre to the SCBU. Bellowa heeded my research recommendation for a minimum acceptable standard of three neonates to one nurse in the SCBU. I had considered that unacceptable neonates-to-nurse ratios were among factors that must be improved upon for Nigeria to achieve her MDG(4) targets. Dr Bellowa was able to deploy more nurses and achieved a patient-to-nurse ratio of 4:1 at the SCBU before the end of his tenure. This was, by far, the best ratio any CMD could achieve in Nigeria during this period. At some other hospital SCBUs, the ratio was as bad as 13:1. He ensured that his six-monthly incubator failure-preventive audit culture (FAC) was meticulously carried out as a matter of priority; this remained unbroken throughout his time in office. NGTH Nguru became one of the best centres in the country with average neonatal mortality rate (NNMR) of 141/1000 presenting neonates as quantified in 2014 – a reduction of nearly 80% from an NNMR of over 680/1000 before the inception of my consultancy at the hospital. Nguru's 2014 record was far better than the national facility-based average of 248/1000 presenting neonates, even without any full-time paediatrician on employment. This seemed to suggest that Nigerian neonates could die more due to lack of appropriate technologies than the absence of highly trained professors or resident medical consultants within the Nigerian rural communities. Nguru performed better than many hospitals with resident consultants; hence the availability of better functional technologies and well-equipped nursing crew were the record-changing factors at play.

The amiable Palati of Suleja

In October 2008, I had just flagged off the incubator project of another tertiary hospital, Abaji Federation Hospital (AFH) Suleja, increasing their SCBU functional incubator capacity from only one to five in a project that took seven days to complete. Hospital management was very pleased with the outcome of the first six months of operation of all five recycled incubator systems. The hospital's Chief Medical Director, Doctor Palati, had been in office about 12 months; however, he was determined to make any possible improvements on neonatal practice outcomes without delay.

When I arrived for a private meeting with Dr Palati, he was still full of excitement over the positive six-month report that had been submitted by the head of his Paediatrics Department concerning the incubators. Very happy and excited, Palati emphasised how it was his dream to make his hospital the best teaching hospital in Nigeria. I could not hide my own happiness at Palati's positive attitude. 'I like your mindset,' I said. 'Just go ahead and dream about it, get like-minded people around you, and I bet you are not far from achieving it.' Dr Palati was very relaxed with my supportive response and my promise to throw in my weight to help him actualise his vision, especially the aspect that related to temperature control in the neonate.

Palati told me more about his dreams and initial frustrations, his strengths and some weaknesses he had inherited from his predecessors in office. He also had the 'awful distractions' from politicians and top Federal Ministry of Health staff to contend with.

'You know what,' said Palati, sitting up suddenly like someone who has just remembered an important point, 'If you have got the time, I will show you what I have had dumped in our stores by some greedy politicians.'

'Yes I do, with all pleasure,' I replied.

Palati took me to a huge store room with various kinds of procured equipment, some wrapped in cellophane and others still in unbroken wooden crates. 'I don't even know what some of these wrapped items are as they were all dumped by politicians as a cover for taking away the funds allocated for the proper running of the hospital,' Palati said sadly.

As we walked past them, I noticed one crate that I suspected could contain an incubator. Palati would not know exactly what was inside, since it was a procurement that was ordered by the preceding hospital management which his Stores Department was yet to sign off to the user department.

'Do you mind if we probe into the contents right away?' I asked.

'Sure, let's see what's in there, shall we?'

Working together, we prised open the top of the crate. 'I knew it! There is definitely an incubator inside,' I exuberantly exclaimed. 'How long has this been here?'

'Not sure, but perhaps up to 12 months or so. I will find out from my stores staff,' said Palati.

The contents of the crate finally turned out to be a top-of-the-range Draeger CALEO incubator system, originally sold by the USA outlet of the German company. Palati discovered that the system had been in the store for 13 months without being installed, due to unresolved issues with the supplier. Even so, the supplier had already been paid the full cost for the supply and installation of the system before the previous hospital management had handed over. Palati and I agreed to allow the hospital's Procurement Department another two months to get the supplier to complete the installation. The given two months was expected to expire on my next trip to Nigeria, after which I, would do it myself. So, after 15 months of storage – by which time the incubator's 12-month warranty had already expired –

the CALEO system was signed off to me for installation at the SCBU.

The previous management of AFH had purchased this state-of-the-art incubator system, but failed to install it, whilst the neonates had continued to die. What were they hiding?

My job now was to install this equipment and also lecture the SCBU staff on its operations and capabilities. I spent plenty of time studying the system's manual and made several long telephone calls to the manufacturers' USA office as indicated in the manual. The Caleo was a super machine that could do a lot for the monitoring of the neonate inside it. Garnished with all kinds of computerised manipulations and artificial intelligence, the Caleo's automatic control system was capable of effective computer decisions for set-point alterations during function. Just like the autopilot in the aviation industry, it was amazing to watch computers gradually take over the making of basic decisions of operational set-point during neonatal incubator care. Any technology enthusiast would be impressed to see the elegance and sophistication of modern top-of-the-range neonatal incubator systems such as the Draeger Caleo.

However, just like an autopilot, medical automation could be deadly without adequate top-quality maintenance. Computer decisions and life-threatening changes come with requirements that must not be compromised during function. The faulty power supply system in Nigeria would not allow the full benefits of incubators like the Caleo. Hence the fundamental operational decisions such as set-point accuracy could become deadly if left to the machine. I wondered if it was reasonable to allow the machine to take over operational decisions of incubator set-point in the Nigerian setting. Servo control techniques were desirable advances, but these were not necessarily safe in Nigeria due to the lack of a good infrastructural support required to operate such technologies. Could application of inappropriate technologies be another reason why the Nigerian neonates died? Absolutely! I referred to many experiences that could support this argument, including an event at the Bida Federal Infirmary (BIFI).

Dr Justus, the Chief Medical Director of BIFI, had invited me to install apnoea monitors at his hospital's Special Care Baby Unit. This was after he had listened to a presentation on how my apnoea monitoring systems were reducing neonatal mortality due to incessant apnoeic attacks. I flew to Abuja and headed to north-west Nigeria via a bumpy road to the small city of Bida. I was welcomed upon arrival by the Paediatrics Department, and was led to the SCBU of the hospital. A radiant-warmer (resuscitaire) system was the first device to be seen as one entered the unit. The resuscitaire was an open warmer device that could also act as a workbench for neonatal treatment, and Nigerian paediatricians often preferred to apply this for monitoring of an unstable neonate. The system had a baby in it at the time of my arrival, and was stationed on the left immediately after the entrance door to the Unit. Dr Segun, the head of the Paediatrics Department, Dr Ada, the clinical head of the SCBU and Mrs Jumo, the ward manager of the SCBU, were all present to welcome me. All four stood beside the entrance door as we chatted. In my characteristic way, my eyes were roving through all functioning equipment and babies in cots within sight as we exchanged greetings.

Suddenly, I spotted a baby on the resuscitaire, observed it

for a while and quickly moved to have a closer look at the baby and the setting of the servo-controlled resuscitaire. The other three professionals followed me. 'Look, this baby must be under massive hyperthermia,' I said, looking Dr Ada in the eye.

'No, it couldn't be. I examined this baby a couple of minutes ago,' replied Dr Ada.

The Matron, Mrs Jumo, agreed with Dr Ada. However, with a smile in my face but still hesitant and looking straight in the eyes of the HOD, I said 'I like to trust my professional judgement'.

Dr Segun, now looking curious, said: 'Certainly; no harm in checking out'. Almost immediately the matron dashed off to check the baby's temperature. Dr Ada went after her while Dr Segun and I continued to chat on. Suddenly the nurses moved in frenzy towards the baby on the resuscitaire, attracting attention. Dr Segun and I moved towards the resuscitaire to join Dr Ada, expecting her to give the update. 'Everything okay?' asked Segun the HOD. 'No, the baby is actually experiencing severe hyperthermia,' Dr Ada replied.

After attending to the baby, Dr Ada asked me, 'But sir, how did you pick up the bad situation just by looking from a distance, without even touching the baby or using any instrument?'

'Years of experience and instinct,' I replied. In the sober voice of professional authority, I continued, 'Actually, attenuation of skin contact with the temperature sensor during servo mode control is a catastrophic factor that is very common in the Nigerian practice. For this reason I do not hesitate to discourage the use of the servo technique for prolonged unattended care of the neonate. Many have died or been made highly morbid due to lack of knowledge of the consequences of skin attenuation'.

Overwhelmed, Dr Ada responded: 'I have never heard of the word 'attenuation' in relation to neonatal temperature control'.

'Yes doctor, I can appreciate that. You can now see that a knowledge gap exists here. Servo technique is not always the best to apply unless one is well aware of this phenomenon and how to avoid it. So, ignorance of such important knowledge is among the reasons why so many neonates have died,' I added.

I initiated an inquiry by sending out a questionnaire to 16 senior consultant paediatricians and chief nursing officers I had met at centres across Nigeria. My question was simple: 'At what incubator set-point do you manage a neonate in your practice'? Surprisingly, I got many different answers. This was a bombshell to me, and I was alarmed. Had I stumbled into an open-ended factor that might have some kind of association with poor neonatal thermoneutral control, and hence high neonatal mortality in Nigeria? There seemed to be no standards here.

An investigation opened up. I made proposals and subsequently collaborated with paediatricians from various parts of Nigeria to embark upon a number of research studies, to understand, from the tropical sub-Saharan perspective, how the incubator set-points might be altered during neonatal care for the best result. These investigations led to the discovery of the 'Handy Approach' technique, which appeared in chapter 28 of the 2012 edition of the Intech global book volume entitled 'Current topics in Tropical Medicine,' edited by Alphonso J RodriguezMorales.

Dr Olaedo, the lady with a heart of gold

Doctor Dugat of Sapele Federal Teaching Hospital was succeeded by another self-styled dynamic CMD, Dr Olaedo. It is very rare to find the kind of dynamism in leadership amongst Nigerian CMDs that Dr Olaedo displayed. Unlike many other successful Nigerian chief executives of federal tertiary Hospitals, she was determined to carry on with most of the laudable programmes that were initiated by Dr Dugat, including the incubator project. Dr Olaedo was a lady with the heart of a lion in her personal determination to successfully carry through her projects irrespective of opposition. No one would be capable of stopping her as she fired on all cylinders in her drive towards the project's completion.

Dr Olaedo's time in office was a period that saw unprecedented development at SFTH. She tried to make the hospital the best in Nigeria, as far as it lay within her powers. Her exuberant character, which often came across as domineering, would land her in the bad books of many of her colleagues after a few years in office. However, any unselfish and patient-friendly practitioner would admire Dr Olaedo's kind-heartedness towards the welfare of patients, bar her last few months in office, when many would have thought otherwise. She favoured no one in her drive to make things work properly. She would quickly refuse any pressure if she was not convinced that a proposal would help her save funds and improve patient care. She often had disagreements and quarrels with me over my style and some dimensions of my work as a visiting consultant to her SCBU. However, the two of us always found a way to move ahead each time for the sake of the poor neonates, sharing the same passion for their survival.

During Olaedo's first two years in office she found it extremely hard to work with me. It was presumed she was still struggling to understand whether my generosity and passion towards the neonates was genuine or not. On one occasion, after a sharp disagreement in her office, I was compelled to give her my resignation letter because of a comment I considered very disrespectful. I considered her comments to have come out of hatred or resentment for my physical appearance and I could not accept or easily pardon that. In the past, I had come across people who made jokes about the way my hair looked, but most people were not bold to make derogatory comments to my face. I was naturally born with soft, loosely-curled hair. This looked very similar to the popular 'Jerry-Curl hair style' that many Nigerian showmen applied to their hair at salons with the use of chemicals. During my university days in Nigeria, people never stopped such questions as: 'why is your hair so curly?' Or 'why do you make yourself look like a showman?' Without feeling offended, I would cheerfully explain that my hair was natural and not the product of chemicals at hair salons. However, quite a few Nigerian people would not bother to ask, but prejudged me for frivolity and hence treated me with contempt. Dr Olaedo might have liked my professional abilities, but this 'vanity look' was unacceptable to her. 'This man could never be a serious fellow with this kind of hairstyle,' she thought.

I felt I had had enough of Olaedo's frequent rejections of my proposals and often snobbish attitude towards me, so I prepared a resignation letter, but I was not sure if it should be submitted because of the poor neonates. A meeting to resolve a simple issue pertaining to my consultancy started to turn sour; perhaps, due to unspoken grudges. As the argument between the two of us continued to get hotter on this occasion, I said: 'CMD, I'm sorry but I won't accept your conditions regarding this issue'. I stood up and excused myself to leave. With a look full of resentment, Dr Olaedo angrily replied, 'You go, who cares? I have got more important things to attend to'. Then in a lower tone but enough for me to hear, she looked up at my hair, then looked down and said, 'I hate fussy guys like you'.

I was about to open the door to leave but the 'fussy guy' comment hit me like a thunderbolt and without any further hesitation, I reached out and pulled the letter from my pocket. I walked back to Olaedo's desk and said: 'Dear CMD, I thank you and the hospital for these years of being a visiting consultant. It has been my pleasure, but I think the time has come to move on.' I handed my resignation letter over to her and left.

As a newly-appointed chief executive, Dr Olaedo was new to the CMDs' club. During the succeeding months, she attended national meetings of the club at Port Harcourt, where she interacted with other CMDs who had benefited so much from my consultancy. She soon understood how genuine my passion for the neonates was as her colleagues showered praises on my contributions. Hence, she began sincere moves for reconciliation, paving the way for me to return to SFTH as a visiting consultant once again.

I hesitated for six months before accepting her invitation. Henceforth Olaedo treated me with great respect, building a very strong friendship that would last her entire seven years in office. She would apply any sentiments to motivate me to assist neonatal practice in her hospital, especially in terms of funding, research and medical devices. Dr Olaedo soon became an influential figure at the CMDs' club. She would do anything to defend my character and personality at national meetings whenever conflicting issues were raised about me. I became a 'dear brother' to her, as she often called me. No one could insult me at any national CMDs' club meetings in Nigeria without incurring the wrath of Dr Olaedo.

I offered regular discounts or donations to Olaedo's SFTH in order to encourage her to continue her collaboration with the nationwide neonatal survival campaign. Like her many other CMD colleagues, Olaedo identified with a number of the strategies I introduced for the reduction of neonatal mortality and adopted these for the Sapele Federal Tertiary Hospital. She embarked on an expansion strategy, increasing her incubator capacity to become the third largest in the country with 24 functional thermoneutral systems. This capacity was built from a fleet of six she inherited from her predecessor in office. Dr Olaedo created a second independent SCBU to specifically cater for babies born within the hospital complex. She passionately favoured the staff training strategy of my consultancy for the development of advanced knowledge on temperature control in the neonate. She insisted on these training courses for her nurses and clinicians, motivating them with promises and awards to acquire this knowledge for better neonatal outcomes. Many of her staff members successfully completed the level 1 course of paediatrics incubation training; many others moved on to level 2, thereby acquiring more essential skills for effective thermoneutral control in the neonate. By the end of 2013 Sapele FTH had won the trophy for the annual national best SCBU awards twice and the runners-up prize also twice. The SCBU became the first in Nigeria to reduce its facility-based neonatal mortality below 80/1000 presenting neonates as compared to the national average that stood at 250/1000 at the time. Her nurses and clinicians became the best in the country in neonatal thermoregulation during incubator care.

This ushered in an era of high success rates as they managed extremely tiny neonates with ease, successfully discharging neonates with birth weights as low as 600 grammes. The other collaborating hospitals in my consultancy were later to catch up with this feat, but by then the Sapele FTH had moved on to higher achievements. Dr Olaedo was a ruthless leader, but I admired her for using her style to achieve great things for neonates at SFTH. The nurses at the SCBU there were assessed as the best in the country in the application of the 'handy approach' technique in the management of very difficult extremely premature neonates (birthweights lower than 1000g or born more than 10 weeks early). On 27th April 2015 – with the use of the handy approach technique – SFTH broke the record for Nigerian hospitals by successfully discharging the tiniest neonate ever, which they nicknamed 'baby Highness'. She was born at a birthweight of 550g at 27 weeks gestation and successfully discharged after 82 days of neonatal nursing. The previous African record at the time was that of baby Victoria, born at a Namibian hospital at 595g birthweight. The SFTH nurses were so good that they repeatedly achieved many months of practice without a single mortality.

The humility of Kumori

At Abiama Federal Infirmary I worked closely with another friend, Dr Kumori, the head of the hospital's neonatal unit. Together, we set up a study protocol to understand why more neonates survived when we strictly applied my newly-devised 'handy-approach', procedures for neonatal thermoneutral control as published in 2012 by Intech in the global book volume entitled 'current topics in tropical medicine'. I later commented: 'This singular application – without any changes to how we treated other appearing morbidities – seemed to have enabled better patient survival for neonates being diagnosed with various diseases. There were drastic reductions in the episodes of neonatal apnoea and the appearance of the morbidities that often instigated apnoea. Our conclusion was that poor neonatal temperature control might be the 'secret factor' that was invariably linked to the inability of neonates to fight back the other conditions being diagnosed'.

Of course, this agreed with the claim that 70-90% of mortality was attributed to low birthweight and prematurity, as most of the neonates so classified would be unable to maintain their physiological body temperatures unassisted. Dr Kumori's SCBU was able to lower their NNMR to 83/1000 presenting neonates as compared to the national facility-based average of 250/1000 in Nigeria, a figure second only to the Sapele Federal Teaching Hospital at the time. Both Kumori and I believed that it was necessary to compare notes in order to fully convince ourselves that lack of adequate thermal stability was the 'force' that weakened the neonates and exacerbated the victories of the various co-morbid factors over them.

Baby Why-Me and Baby Not-Me

My teammates and I were becoming more and more aware of the successes we could achieve if neonates were prevented from acquiring body temperatures outside the physiological limits (i.e. 36.5°C – 37.4°C). This was just what the 'handy-approach' was used for. Continuous practical demonstration of the technique during the days of my consultancy at any SCBU became vital in order to ensure that all nurses and clinicians learnt how to apply the flowchart. I would normally do my ward-rounds with the nurses to identify the very difficult cases, especially amongst the premature, low-birthweight and extremely low-birthweight neonates. I would choose one or two of the neonates, mainly the most vulnerable, to designate as my handy-approach 'case neonates' during each consultancy visit. This was often a period of about seven days during my six-monthly visit to each SCBU. The clinicians and nurses were free to continue to attend to the case neonates as usual, except for temperature control and incubator manipulation. These were strictly reserved for me to carry out under the watch of all clinicians and nurses present as they learnt how the handy approach was implemented on the various presenting conditions of the neonate.

The story of a child I will call 'baby Why-Me' was a tragic example that demonstrated the efficiency of my handy approach at Edo Federal Infirmary. Why-Me was born at the hospital with an extremely low birthweight of 650g and had been managed at the SCBU for six days before I arrived for my six-monthly routine visit. The neonate's condition was continuously declining from the day of admission. The baby was experiencing up to eight episodes of apnoea daily and the doctors had advised the parents that their baby might never recover. They were literally waiting for baby to give up at any moment as its weight had dropped to 490g by the sixth day of its life. Doctors gave the baby another 24 hours to live. When I reviewed the case, all odds were against its survival, until I noticed that the baby had never experienced consistent safe body temperature for up to six hours since admission. I pointed out to the medical team that it was not correct to abandon the baby's life until it had been sustainably kept stable within the thermal safe-zone temperatures. 'This is more dependent on the skills of the practitioner than the will of the neonate to survive,' I said.

I adopted the baby as my practise 'case neonate' for the seven-day visit, asking all nurses and resident doctors on duty to always report to the neonate's incubator as I implemented the dynamics of thermoneutral stabilisation using the handy-approach technique. Within the succeeding three-hour period, the technique enabled the baby's body temperature to be controlled, driving it into the physiological thermal safe zone of 36.5°C – 37.4°C. I continued the half-hourly process of ensuring that the baby's stability was maintained as the nurses learnt this process. They passed information to their colleagues from one nursing shift to the next. I continued to direct the process through telephone calls whenever I was not present on the ward.

The first pleasant surprise to be noticed by the nursing and clinical crew after 24 hours was that the baby's apnoeic frequency had reduced by 50% as compared to the preceding three days. I also imposed another exceptional rule on baby's management that allowed only one nurse in every shift to attend to the baby. 'We had previously used this method at the Abiama Federal Infirmary to minimise the chances of transferring microorganisms from stronger neonates to weaker ones,' I explained. This would happen imperceptibly because the often overworked nurses rarely washed their hands or changed their gloves in between attending to other stronger patients.

The incidence of infection reduced amongst this class of neonates when I tested this method, involving fewer or specifically assigned nurses. 'We must guard baby Why-Me from any possible infection at this stage as this could spell disaster,' I warned during a meeting with the Ward Manager. Baby Why-Me was now turning into a special patient as his body temperature had been very stable for three days and apnoeic attacks had stopped. The baby's feeding normalised without the frequently occurring regurgitation which had previously exacerbated the situation. Baby's body weight had not dropped any further from 490g. However, I noticed that thermoneutral control was beginning to indicate a need for gradual reduction in the incubator set-point for the maintenance of the baby's thermal requirement as compared to the day of its conscription as my case neonate. On the first day, the incubator needed to run at full body temperature of 36.9°C to achieve baby's thermal stability; however, by the fourth day this was now running at 36.1°C. This was a clear indication that baby was beginning to respond by making little contributions towards its body heat requirement.

After the morning ward round and review of baby Why-Me's progress, I said to the team of nurses and doctors: 'Every factor

I have considered important in this case looks very promising to me. If we continue as we have done so far, ensuring that this baby is protected from infection, baby will definitely gain its initial weight within the next 48 hours.'

Strangely, there was no show of excitement from the nurses after my prediction. I followed the matron, Mrs Orobo, to her office and said to her: 'Matron, you expressed surprise that this baby is still alive, but why did you people show no signs of excitement at my predictions of weight gain?'

'Doctor, the prediction was too good to be easily acceptable,' she replied. 'It is thrilling enough that baby is still alive. However, if weight gain is ever achieved after these many days of continuous deterioration, then it will be an obvious wonder. My colleagues did not really believe you based on our past experiences. This is why you did not get the reaction you expected, sorry.'

'What if baby gains weight as I predicted?' I asked.

'Weight gain? That would be walking into a new era,' replied Matron Orobo.

I carefully arranged to continue my routine on the case neonate for vital signs checks and instructions for thermo-regulation of the incubator; this continued as usual through telephone calls when I was away from the ward. By this arrangement, Matron Orobo would provide me with data updates of vital signs over the phone. In the morning of the 13th day of baby's life, I was at my hotel room getting ready to depart to Owerri to start at my next hospital on schedule, the Owerri Federal Teaching Hospital. My phone rang and it was Matron Orobo calling.

'Hello matron, I hope everything is fine with baby Why-Me?' I asked.

'Oh yes, doctor,' Matron Orobo began, 'Doctor, wonders shall never end! Baby weighed 500 grams this morning, gaining 10 grams exactly as you predicted. Baby has remained quite stable, thermally and otherwise and feeding well. We were all amazed and excited this morning. Every person here wishes you a safe trip on your journey.'

'Great news,' I replied. 'Please continue with the good work and keep me updated'.

I continued my routine updating with baby Why-Me for the next seven days. Matron Orobo and her team seemed to have appreciably understood this routine and now had little need of my advice. Baby continued its weight gain on a daily basis until it weighed 710 g on its 20th day of life, seven days after its first weight gain. This was the day I was scheduled to leave Owerri for the Tertiary Hospital of Enugu. Later that day, I called Matron Orobo: 'Matron I think you have done very well so far with your team and I must encourage you to continue the good work,' I said. 'I am now relocating to another hospital and will soon be heading to northern Nigeria and may not be calling for daily updates any more. However, do not hesitate to alert me whenever you particularly need my input, please. If all things continue as they are presently, baby will definitely weigh more than 1000 grams within the next two weeks. Please maintain the standards and do everything necessary to prevent this baby from infection, because it might still not survive that.'

The news of baby Why-Me's turnaround spread like wildfire within the department, reviving every hope of the baby's survival. Its parents were very hopeful and thankful. They pestered Matron Orobo to assist them to contact me on the phone so as to say 'thank you'. They stopped at nothing with matron Orobo until they spoke personally with me, whilst I was consulting at another SCBU in northern Nigeria. I applied the data from baby Why-Me's file whilst delivering a lecture session at my current SCBU in the north. The lecture had barely ended when my phone rang and the caller introduced himself as the father of the tiny patient at Edo hospital. He was very thankful, expressing his gratitude to God for bringing me to the hospital at the right time for their baby. They were already beginning to celebrate baby's survival.

But then, tragedy struck. It was Friday night, and the baby's oxygen respiratory support was continuing. Unknown to the SCBU staff, this was the last oxygen cylinder available. This kind of failure was typical of hospitals in Nigeria – going into three days of weekend services unprepared for emergencies such as the need for oxygen. So the oxygen finished after midnight on Friday without standby oxygen set in the ward. Baby Why-Me suffered a serious setback, compounded by a power cut that turned off the incubator for several hours before morning time. Shamefully, it took many hours of no power, exacerbating the risks of hypothermia and hypoxia owing to lack of oxygen before day came and the father could go in search of oxygen by himself in the city, although many shops had closed for the weekend. Baby Why-Me had also remained hypothermic for many hours as the few nurses on weekend duty tried to assist the baby by wrapping it with cloth next to a hot water bottle to keep warm. This was not enough for thermal stabilization, and so this weekend crisis started a catastrophe that would soon end baby Why-Me's life after all that struggle.

By the time work resumed on Monday morning when more experienced staff were on duty, baby Why-Me had already turned into a 'living vegetable'. Matron Orobo phoned me to report the events of the weekend: 'I am also sorry that I noticed some yellowish discharges from baby's nose this morning and doctors have just confirmed baby has developed some kind of infection. Baby has also remained weak and we are finding it difficult to thermally stabilize it due to apnoea that has started re-occurring at short intervals,' she said.

I was devastated and remained sad all day. Unfortunately, the ultimate bad news arrived as matron later phoned again to confirm that baby Why-Me had passed away in the early hours of Tuesday.

The sad case of baby Why-Me was an eye opener that strengthened my argument that temperature control should be given the highest priority in neonatal care. It became desirable for me to initiate a formal research investigation on this topic, but I needed preliminary evidence to establish a good hypothesis. Right across all my collaborating hospitals, Owerri, Kano, Benin City, Abuja, Lagos, Enugu, Yola, Nguru, etc., I watched for opportunities among the best presenting cases. I intensified my motivation for the management of the hospitals to support my campaign for more SCBU nurses and doctors to enrol for my paediatrics incubation courses to improve their neonatal temperature control skills. Many doctors enthusiastically enrolled, and the nurses were ever more willing to acquire this skill as they perceived that they were realising better outcomes from case neonates whenever I was around during my consulting visits.

The story of baby Why-Me and the data extracted from the case file were used in running my nationwide training courses across Nigeria. The matron of the SCBU at Oriaku Federal Tertiary Hospital (OFTH) said to me at the completion of the course series: 'This subject is difficult, but we would like to make a deliberate effort in my unit to prevent outcomes such as baby Why-Me. We would prefer 'baby Not-Me''.

Within two days of completing the course at OFTH, the SCBU admitted an extremely low birthweight neonate of 650g and 27 weeks of gestation (GA). This was in addition to an earlier admission of a 750g, 28-week GA neonate on the same day. At about the same period, the outborn SCBU of the hospital was already managing another baby of 700g BW. The Outborn SCBU ward was dedicated to babies that were not delivered at OFTH but rather referred from other facilities. This was a standard Nigerian practice at the tertiary level that ensured the minimisation of cross-infection from such outside-born patients. So in between the two SCBUs, test and control case scenarios dramatically set themselves in place for comparative investigation. The 750g and 700g neonates died within 48 hours of their admission. This was expected because they were managed following SCBU's usual practice procedure. It was uncommon at the time for extremely low birthweight neonates, below 800g, to survive at OFTH. However, Matron Mary of Inborn SCBU assigned the best two members of her team to carefully follow the handy-approach technique to exclusively manage the 650g neonate. The two nurses were chosen based on the perception that they were ahead of the rest in their level of understanding of the technique. This neonate, being much small than the other two, was expected to die as well. This assumption, however, turned out wrong as baby survived the first seven days and went on to be successfully discharged. Baby Not-Me became a highly celebrated case, as it was the first time OFTH would successfully discharge such a tiny neonate. Inborn SCBU officially nicknamed the neonate 'Baby Not-Me' after the seventh day of its life.

In her excitement, Matron Mary said to me: 'Doctor, we can confidently say that you are right and the handy approach works. We did it, but it is still a great surprise to all of us. We never altered any other management technique bar temperature control as prescribed by the handy approach flowchart, so we do not need to panic any more at the appearance of such extremely tiny or premature neonates as we can really help them. Indeed temperature control is the key.'

The hospital subsequently accepted my proposals to install two parallel sets of power banking systems (PBS) to provide uninterrupted power to serve the incubators during power cuts. The CMD of the hospital, on getting this report from the nurses, said to me: 'I so much appreciate your heroism in championing our excellent neonatal outcomes. I will personally lead the motivational campaign for my staff to enrol on the courses you deliver during your visits in order to improve on these fantastic results.'

CHAPTER 9

THE 'CATERPILLARS' AT WORK

✦✦✦✦✦✦✦

The battle to define and eradicate the major factors responsible for high neonatal mortality would have been a lot easier for my growing team of like-minded associates if it had not been for some people who tried to thwart me with premeditated intentions to frustrate all my efforts. If these people had known that their greed, wickedness and ill-motivated desire to fight against a course they felt did not gratify them would eventually contribute to the colossal failure of the 'millennium development goal,' they would perhaps have behaved differently. Unfortunately, their actions were the major impediments to progress. My rather crazy attempts to save the teeming population of dying neonates against the monstrously evil tide of these materialistic caterpillars, coupled with the high risks of the Nigerian bad roads full of terrorists and kidnappers, unavailability of functional infrastructure to enable effective services and all kinds of disabling problems with potentials of crippling any good ideas, can be likened to a 'rescue operation in a stormy sea'. My life and those of the few young people that worked with me at various times were at constant high risk. My body system functioned on high adrenaline like a soldier on the fiercest battle front. Every success scored was like 'victory from a blizzard'.

The battle of terrified technicians

The engineering and maintenance departments of Nigerian hospitals had a huge task to ensure that all technical systems were operational at all times. This was a difficult job to do, as many of them were ill-qualified as system engineers or designers. Maintenance workshops and work attitudes were full of all kinds of safety hazards. Most of the staff did not understand the international codes of safe practice for medical devices; some confessed of lack of awareness of any such codes and practices. The in-house engineers, as they were sometimes called at the hospitals, were engulfed with desire to make some private money out of any equipment they managed to fix. They inflated the cost of spare parts or made financial requests for money for components that were not needed, all in an attempt to defraud the hospitals. Huge sums of money were often demanded so as to be enough to be shared amongst all interested parties based on an agreed formula for each job. Management staff other than the technicians were sometimes involved. These shameful acts were often performed to the detriment of the patients whose lives depended on the functionality of the faulty systems. One wonders why these 'educated illiterates', as I often called them, found it hard to understand that their monthly salaries were the pay for the jobs they carried out. If an external contractor or a specialist engineer were to take up a job that the in-house engineers could not handle, then this contractor was forced to agree on some sharing formula before the contract award could be supported by the staff of Works Department. The technicians never bothered much about the capabilities of contractors; jobs could be awarded to contractors with little experience provided they were willing to connive in this unethical practice with them. Very often, fully paid-for jobs could be uncompleted or poorly executed without questions being asked because the staff involved had sophisticated methods of covering up frauds of this nature. It was except in a very few instances, to find contractors who insisted on decent practice and high standards of safety.

Many of the technicians from these hospitals were very uncomfortable with the standards I exhibited, as it was difficult for them to implement their shameful acts with me. In truth, I was there to execute a specialist job, well known to be too technical for the in-house engineers, yet they sought to be paid bribes or to get the cost of the job increased to accommodate the cash they wanted to get out of the job. Some were bold enough to open up such discussions with me; others used body language to pass the information for fear of being quoted. The saddest aspect of this was that the effective restoration of the faulty systems did not matter much to these gullible people compared to the extra cash they diverted into their private pockets. Some tried to befriend or bully me to win me over; but when they could not achieve this, they opted to label me an enemy and resorted to blackmail. Unfortunately for them, my neonatal solutions were so uniquely effective that the blackmails were often ignored by CMDs, who refused to terminate my consultancy. They would rather keep the consultancy in order to maintain an operationally manageable SCBU.

At some hospitals, the in-house technicians and engineers felt threatened and fought back at what they saw as somebody coming to take over their jobs and making them look unintelligent, preventing their unlawful manoeuvres and still refusing their proposals for cash gratification. I never hesitated to tender my resignation to the few hospital managements that dared accept, defend or support the blackmails from technicians. This however never helped matters as following my withdrawal at each centre, the systems soon begin to shut down owing to lack of proper maintenance, and the neonates' death rate would soar again.

Iyang, a systems maintenance technician at Lafia Federal Infirmary (LFI), was forced to admit that he was still relevant and capable of doing the specialist jobs that I was regularly invited to do for the hospital. I had been a visiting consultant on thermoneutral devices at the hospital for the last three years of the immediate-past CMDs, Doctor Dulami and Doctor Rapin. The SCBU was routinely maintained at a negotiated contract sum without any gratification to any group of hospital staff or individuals, as usual with me. Uninterrupted system functionality and minimised failures at the Unit brought about unprecedentedly high neonatal survival at the SCBU during this period. Some individuals were unhappy at the lack of financial gratification from me. They were led by a senior staff member of the Procurement Department named Ibram. Mr Ibram teamed up with some like-minded 'caterpillars' from the Works and Accounts Departments to frame me to get rid of me. They first tried blackmail to force me into giving them regular 'cuts' from my pay. They mounted pressure on the newly-appointed CMD, who was completely oblivious of all the previous SCBU disasters that had led to my invitation and consultancy at the Unit. A self-confessed righteous man, the new CMD, Dr Pumsha, fell into their trap. After assuming office, he decided to go all out to witch-hunt his immediate past predecessor for any indictable evidence in order to settle some previous scores with him. He began to scrutinize all contracts awarded by Dr Dulami, who was arguably a better person than the self-righteous Dr Pumsha. He questioned the authenticity of my passion for neonatal survival, especially as there was a cordial relationship between Dulami and me. Pumsha was a church deacon, but his heart was full of hatred against the neonatal programme, perhaps for selfish reasons. His actions slowed the SCBU progress as though Satan used him as an agent for the deaths of many neonates at the Lafia hospital. Pumsha soon fell to the hands of the gullible seekers of gratification and never bothered about the lives of the poor neonates.

He summoned Mr Iyang, the technician, demanding to explain why he was not technically as good as Dr Hippolite. Dr Pumsha wanted to know why Iyang must be on employment whilst the hospital paid a consultant to do an aspect of the job he presumably had been employed to do. Dr Pumsha was a typical 'educated' Nigerian medical consultant, who would normally think it was okay to demand an ordinary technician to achieve the same professional feats as the highly-educated Hippolite.

Pumsha threatened to fire Mr Iyang for not being as good as me: a non-graduate technician to be like a Royal London PhD medical engineer! Pumsha was unreal. He was a disgrace to both Christianity and the medical profession on the account of this demand. Of course, Mr Iyang was afraid and did not want to lose his job, so he had to claim to Pumsha that it was a waste of funds keeping me on consultancy.

'Sir, I can effectively do all the jobs for which this Hippolite was being paid lots of money by the two previous CMDs,' Iyang stated.

'What percent of this contract sum was Hippolite giving to the last CMD for him to have been there for so long?' Pumsha asked.

'I do not know sir, but he might be giving something to the past CMD as his pay was too much for the sort of work he did,' answered Iyang.

Dr Pumsha was pleased with Iyang's answers. This meant terminating my agreement with the hospital. Actually, I saw this coming and assisted Pumsha to hasten it by submitting my resignation letter ahead of our final meeting on the matter. What happened next was neonatal disaster after disaster. Mr Iyang could not cope, so the SCBU crashed so badly that parents threatened to take the hospital to court due to mismanaged neonatal cases. There were sad newspaper articles such as the one shown in News Appendix 2 – (warning: the hospital's real name has been obscured). Characters like Dr Pumsha and Mr

Iyang were enemies of the Nigerian healthcare system and represented more reasons why the Nigerian neonates died.

In a related incident at Kamalu Federal Teaching Hospital, the story was similar. The chief technician, Mr Nyaku, blackmailed Dr Abayomi, the immediate past CMD, in order to gain the admiration of Dr Brown, the newly appointed CMD, so as to get rid of me. Mr Nyaku got what he wanted when Brown began to question if it was really necessary to involve an outside consultant in a job his in-house team claimed they could do. Brown eventually frustrated me, for which I later tendered my resignation and withdrew my consultancy. What happened next? As you may guess, over the succeeding three years, the SCBU gradually deteriorated, losing its functional incubators, and eventually crashed to a halt in the fourth year. It got so bad that the consultant clinician in charge of the SCBU decided to shut down the entire unit, challenging the management: 'it is impossible for us to run a SCBU without functional incubators'. So, for the love of dirty cash these men sent countless neonates to untimely graves.

Some of these indirect neonatal murderers are still among the self-confessed righteous men seen parading themselves as 'honourable' people in Nigeria today. It is understood that most of these people do not often realise how much their actions contribute towards neonatal deaths. The crisis that soon engulfed the CMD and the KFTH was an embarrassment to the Federal Ministry of Health. It was so bad that the CMD quickly realised that he had been deceived, and hence had to find a way to fix things in order to save his job. He soon realised that the return of my consultancy was inevitable if the visiting probe team from FMoH were not to find the SCBU in its then dysfunctional state. The CMD made haste to re-establish contact and pleaded with me to resume my terminated consultancy. This was after over three years of running down all my initial achievements at the SCBU.

It was such a shame for Mr Nyaku and the men of his Works Department when I arrived to resume my consultancy after over three years of being rejected. They had no choice when, at my demand, the CMD banned Mr Nyaku and his gang from touching any thermoneutral system at the SCBU. Dr Brown, or should I say the hospital, had some financial punishment to attend to before my acceptance to intervene. I demanded a condition that required them to pay the sum of ₦450,000 they owed me, which Nyaku had made the hospital refuse to pay at the time my consultancy was terminated. In addition, I demanded the accruable interest on this amount at 29% APR compounded over four years, similar to my credit card conditions. I also demanded an upfront payment of 80% cost of the proposed restoration works. The resulting amount was huge, but Dr Brown did not hesitate in paying it. It was a time of shame for Mr Nyaku.

Mr Nyaku was not a good man. After all indictments, no one was punished, even after many babies had been so recklessly murdered. The blood of those babies cries from their graves, because they died of preventable causes and through the wrongful actions of people such as Mr Nyaku.

Comparable incidences happened at many other federal teaching hospitals and medical centres at various times around the country – Enugu, Abakaliki, Calabar, Sokoto, Lagos, Benin City, Owerri, Gwagwalada, and Kano, just to mention a few.

I refused them all, resisted them all and conquered them all to defend the new-born babies.

Undermining the nursing management culture

Experienced paediatric specialist nurses were massively in short supply in Nigeria. This was reflected in the scarcity of trained neonatal specialist nurses across all tertiary hospitals. It was a nightmare to manage large number of neonates in the absence of adequate pre-qualified personnel. The nursing departments of the Nigerian tertiary hospitals were powerful sub-units of the hospital management, usually headed by the Director of Nursing Services. The DNS reported directly to the Chief Medical Director, who of course was usually more powerful than the entire hospital institution itself. The CMD could wake up or with one command destroy or run down such a huge institution with the consequence of many deaths, and bribe himself out of the mess without any punishment. The Nigerian Nursing Services Directorate had a culture of compulsory periodic rotation, or shuffling all nursing staff around the various departments or patient units of the hospital, irrespective of their areas of specialisation. By this culture, a paediatric trained nurse could be posted to work in an orthopaedic trauma ward whilst the hospital had a massive shortage of paediatric nurses – madness! Some hospitals carried out this reshuffling as frequent as every two years, or even annually. A highly specialised ward like the SCBU ought to have adequate nurses with special skills tailored to the management of the newborn in order to succeed. They must have the skills to understand or interpret many neonatal characteristics and signs, including crying in different circumstances. I would often talk about my vast experience: 'In my research investigations, I discovered that the most important aspect of these essential skills for neonatal care was thermoneutral control, which meant maintaining the neonate's body temperature within its physiological limits, 36.5°C to 37.4°C, and practising with full infection-control consciousness, especially during the first seven days of life'. These two factors were found to contribute 55% and 30% of the neonatal death burden recorded in Nigerian facilities, respectively. This was to say that four in every five neonates who would die in a Nigerian facility within the first seven days of life would have been adversely affected by poor temperature control or infection of various kinds.

Sadly I never witnessed any new nurse arriving at my SCBUs, either freshly employed or from a reshuffling exercise, with an acceptable knowledge level of these two crucial factors. The nurse reshuffling exercise almost always left the SCBU as an experimentation ward, where the lives of innocent tiny babies were left in the hands of inexperienced nurses. Mistakes, negligence and outright ignorance were common, and many neonates died as a result of this pointless practice. The Nursing Directorate would not give up the practice as they used it to 'train' or give other nurses the 'experience' of working in the other aspects of nursing care. I, however, maintained that the neonates were too vulnerable to be so used. I would solicit for the intervention of the CMDs. I fought against this practice, though with successes which were few and often did not last beyond the remaining period of time an intervening CMD had to stay in office. I insisted that the reshuffling exercise must not affect any neonatal certified nurse or more than 10% of the remaining SCBU-experienced nurses at the same time.

The restraining order worked in some hospitals, but only whilst the incumbent CMD remained. Soon ill-motivated nurses challenged the order under a new DNS or CMD and had the neonatal preferential treatment dismantled. After this kind of exercise came weeks and months of the incessant cries of bereaved mothers as their precious babies die at the hands of 'learner nurses' in the SCBU. The weekly and monthly mortality reports revealed these anomalies, yet DNSs still loved to practise their parochial ideas. This insensitive practice was another reason why so many Nigerian babies had died.

The practical demonstrations and documentation of data at the various hospitals where I consulted convinced the nurses and clinicians that the new techniques and procedures I was introducing were actually improving neonatal survival at their SCBUs. The clinicians and nurses could recite theories of what was generally believed, and the opinions of foreign authors concerning African neonates and their high mortality rates. Knowledge of the high neonatal mortality rate and their so-called causes were repeatedly being recycled in scientific journals by Nigerian authors. Why fill scientific journals with repetition?

Doctor Kumbi, a senior doctor, has been notified that he is due for promotion assessment in 12 months. He picks up the phone and begins to call all his friends, including Dr Okukpo: 'Can you include my name as co-author in that paper you are writing?' 'Okay, no problem, consider it done, sir,' responds Dr Okukpo. He goes ahead and includes Kumbi as a co-author of a piece of scientific research that Kumbi knew nothing about, let alone having the ability to defend its findings. Dr Kumbi goes on appending his name to all sorts of journal papers without getting involved in the work himself, and soon he accumulates enough for the next promotion. On and on Dr Kumbi climbs, up to the position of 'professor' in a scientific field without any legacy of championing an impactful study that makes a proper addition to knowledge. This is the Nigeria academia. They will repeatedly highlight contributory causes of neonatal mortality: septicaemia and pneumonia 50%, birth asphyxia 20%, prematurity 20% and congenital malformation 10%, and such like. Whenever my computer flagged up a new publication on Nigerian neonates, I would hope that a new discovery or possible solution might have been found. However, the paper is soon revealed to be another repetition of already known problems or the same statistical information about incidences at a location or hospital, and hence remains empty of fresh useful information. So many publications, but still no hope for the neonates!

Most of the neonatal mortalities happened amongst low birthweight (LBW) infants; in fact up to 70-90% of deaths were LBW and extremely LBW infants. Information such as this was recited by student doctors to pass exams. The backward-looking academic system blocked the creative minds of the young students and the ability of young doctors to think afresh, to research into deeper meanings of these statistics amongst the dying neonates.

I wanted to know all about this information and why so much seemed to be known, but the neonatal mortality rate was not falling. During one of my medical mission trips in Nigeria, I was chatting with one of my friends, an experienced professor of paediatrics, Professor Olusa, from the north-west Nigeria about this monster of high NNMR. I asked him: 'why does it seem so much is known about NNMR, its causes and management, yet poor practice outcome is as common in Nigeria as the very paediatrics profession?'

'I am also ashamed of this and we might be right to think we have been putting too much of our energies in the wrong direction and so our efforts were not achieving good results,' Olusa replied.

Olusa was an open-minded professional who was eager to join my team to synthesize a new approach of looking at the whole NNMR problem in Nigeria. I did a lot of literature searching, studying many journal articles relating to NNMR from Nigerian authors, these being numerous between 1990 and 2010, the millennium development goal years. I desperately searched the journal articles for solutions that must have been discovered and forgotten, but I was disappointed. I eagerly sought to isolate the articles with clearly defined and validated solutions that were tailored to Nigeria's high NNMR reduction, separating these from articles that merely reported or repeated the incidences, prevalence or perceived causes of this problem from different parts of the country. I was disappointed to realise that less than 2% of all the articles made any attempt at introducing an in-country validated problem-solving idea, most just re-emphasising the existence of the problem from different institutions or parts of the country. The academic researcher upon whose shoulders the discoveries required for lowering NNMR rested were more interested in academic titles and promotion than the ordeals of neonates. They never lost sleep for the sake of the dying babies but for the sake of delayed salaries and promotions. The neonates died because they never bothered.

CHAPTER 10

FRUSTRATION, APATHY AND ENVY

✦✦✦✦✦✦✦

I made a lot of friends amongst the doctors and nurses I came across in my work as I covered the whole of Nigeria, giving equal opportunity to every Nigerian neonate irrespective of tribe and religion. To me, every neonate mattered, whether born in the city or in the most inaccessible places.

However, later events gave clear proof that some of my supposed friends were unhappy that I was achieving such success with my unconventional approach, and hence stealing the attention away from them. This impression might be wrong, but such was my feeling at times of interview. There were no such impressions from most of the colleagues that researched and published with me. A very senior Nigerian paediatrician encouraged me on several occasions, saying she was aware how envious some colleagues had become of my success: 'Many of our colleagues are making life difficulty for you just because of envy,' she said. 'Please do not mind them, but remain focused for the sake of the neonates.' I felt that the situation was made worse by the fact that I was primarily an engineer and not a first-degree medical doctor. Unfortunately, a lot of Nigerian doctors felt superior to other professionals. This egotism might, in part, be understandable, as university admission to study medicine in Nigeria was extremely tough and more competitive than other fields of study, so, there was a lot of pride associated with admission to study medicine, which often lasted all through the period of study. Sometimes I wondered why some of these friends were still happy to clog my progress towards this important goal for the nation – especially those that had known me from the very difficult beginning of my medical career.

I once said to one of those old neonatologist friends, Dr Ojuku: 'With all the convincing preliminary evidence from your SCBUs, I think we may have to formally initiate a comparative investigative study based on the hypothesis that temperature control is responsible for most of the neonatal deaths involving premature babies in Nigeria. Our study-control data would be based on retrospective cases to be extracted from your data bank at the Records Department of the hospital'.

Unlike many other paediatricians I had worked with, Dr Ojuku did not show any sign of excitement at the proposal; he rather resorted to quizzing me on my level of understanding of the immediate postnatal physiology of a neonate. The rhetorical questions were as though my friend was trying to examine me for an MB BS degree exam. I hid my sad feelings and humbly tried to explain what I knew to the best of my practised knowledge. Dr Ojuku continued to show off with further questions: 'At what stage after birth do you think temperature becomes a critical issue?' he asked. 'Okay, my dear friend Ojuku, it may vary from case to case but be it whenever it might, we have a clear hypothesis here and this is what I propose for us to investigate,' I responded. 'If you are interested, just say so and we shall be on the move. Together, we shall learn from our investigation and then teach others for the good of the neonates to come then after.'

This superiority complex would not let the doctor have any meaningful discussion with me. One would have thought that being a Royal University London PhD in such a rare academic field would compel him to show some respect and treat me differently. 'I will think about your proposal and get back to you,' concluded Dr Ojuku.

The Chief Medical Director of the hospital earnestly wanted me to execute this research at her centre, but Dr Ojuku was unaware of the CMD's interest. The long wait for a definite answer from Ojuku rather upset the CMD. Dr Ojuku dragged this on for another six months before his CMD decided to intervene. She requested another younger female consultant in the department to collaborate and get the study started. With the support of the CMD, the younger consultant made her initial moves to obtain some archived files from the Records Department. When Dr Ojuku discovered this move, he confronted the consultant and questioned why she should reveal any clinical data to an outsider, referring to me.

'Did you say 'an outsider'?' questioned the younger consultant. Dr Ojuku did not respect the fact that I was an officially appointed visiting consultant to the Unit who had brought in a lot of record-breaking successes for the centre. The younger consultant, unwilling to fight for whatever rights she might have, decided to opt out of the research study to avoid further confrontations with Dr Ojuku.

I was very disappointed and felt insulted at Dr Ojuku's behaviour and for considering me an 'outsider'. Was Dr Ojuku envious of me? If not, why the resentment and verbal insults? He was well aware that I had been a legitimate visiting consultant to the hospital's SCBU for over five years, and that I was the key person who had initiated the very good results the SCBU was celebrating.

The CMD was already aware of what was going on before I could officially complain to her. As we discussed the matter, I said: 'CMD, I have nearly 15 other Nigerian tertiary hospitals in my consultancy as you are well aware of, and I can easily initiate this scientific investigation at another SCBU somewhere else around the country where I am better appreciated. However, being one of the foremost Nigerian hospitals in the application of this new technique, and as you have worked so hard to motivate your staff for this, I felt your hospital is the most justifiable centre to carry out this study and to claim the praise that would be associated with the work after journal publication. Sadly, with all these ugly events and the insults from Dr Ojuku, I have decided to turn to another hospital for this investigation. Sorry.'

The CMD was disappointed at my decision and apologised. I wondered how unfortunate Dr Ojuku's character had been and wished he had behaved differently. 'Professional apathy and intolerance are among the reasons why so many neonates have died,' I said to the CMD and left.

At one of the tertiary hospitals in north-west Nigeria, I observed another knowledge gap on phototherapy application and wished to initiate an investigative research study. The study proposal I developed was readily acceptable to an apparent friend who was a senior clinical staff member of the SCBU. She jumped at the idea, exclaiming: 'Wow, it will be great to carry out this study; I am definitely interested'. Dr Omacha's enthusiasm was understandable, as the resulting publication would definitely enhance her chances of the academic promotion that people in her current position desired most. I realised much later that some Nigerian academics loved my resilience and research skills and what I could professionally offer, but definitely not my personality, sadly. It was also sad that many of the senior Nigerian medical consultants and professors in such busy units as the SCBU were hardly around during consulting hours to personally guide their resident students. They were often too busy with activities and engagements outside their hospitals, travelling all over the country and overseas, often leaving their medical students to learn by 'trial and error' using poor innocent neonates.

It was necessary for me to persuade my clinician friend to appoint one of her resident students to anchor the proposed research study for data collection. I reasoned that this would minimise the frustrations I would encounter trying to pursue the senior consultant around on her 'never-in-town' travel engagements. An easy motivation would be to find a way of making this investigation the student's official fellowship project. Initially, the proposal sounded good to Dr Omacha, so based on my suggestion, she agreed to develop a tailored abstract capable of making the proposal a generally acceptable one for the Medical Postgraduate College of Nigeria.

I expected Dr Omacha to harmonise the research question so that it could fit into the standard structure of the Nigerian Postgraduate Medical College for acceptance. I said to her: 'It is always easy to fit the stereotype, but people that blaze the trail must be prepared for extra work outside the box'. My dream was to apply research techniques to investigate unclear phenomena around SCBUs, and to infuse the findings into the conventional management of neonates in order to create some unconventional techniques that might help improve survival.

Dr Omacha was too busy as usual, so she was unable to modify my write-up into an acceptable proposal for the resident doctor she wished to select as the anchor person for the research. She simply filed the raw draft proposal I gave to her and hence failed to secure the acceptance. I was disappointed, but not because of the rejection of the proposal. Dr Omacha could have delivered the bad news with some humility, or have expressed her shame for failing to produce an acceptable research proposal. Instead she rather preferred to make comments that tended to castigate my 'engineering approach'. She was happy to accept the co-authorship of the previous work I had carried out because these had added to her quest for publications that could enhance her academic promotion. She wanted this, whether she had little or nothing to contribute to the research. However, when it was down to doing the dirty work, she forgot the neonates for whom I laboured and rather claimed that I applied 'engineering methods that were not acceptable in medicine'. What nonsense! Dr Omacha declared like an absolute matriarch: 'It is not possible to assign this project to one of our students as it is not a clinical project'. Surprised and bewildered, I asked: 'And so what is it when it addresses clinical issues in the neonate?'

'This is an engineering project and not suitable for a doctor to execute, however we can still conduct the investigation for journal publication only,' she replied.

Annoyed at this declaration I said: 'I am surprised that the high neonatal mortality rate in Nigeria is not a clinical problem to Nigerian clinicians like you, since the synthesis of a solution for this is not a clinical project to you. I would appreciate it if you can give me some time to think about your 'publication only' interest.'

Unknown to Dr Omacha, I had already had enough of this kind of behaviour and unconcerned attitude of the supposed custodians of neonatal health in Nigeria. This made me, there and then, decide never to carry out any further joint research with Dr Omacha. I continued with my research with many other consultants across Nigeria, but avoided paediatricians like Dr Omacha. She would frantically request me to enlist her in the many other publications that followed but I would always explain that 'the nature of the research was not clinical enough' to accommodate her class of practice, hoping she would understand what I meant. This kind of behaviour still continues to deny the Nigerian neonate the synthesis of useful solutions that could guarantee their survival.

There were still many practitioners who had deep concerns for neonatal failures in Nigeria. These individuals were humble enough to team up for whatever solution could help. The SCBU of Lafiaji Federal Hospital was another neonatal unit that was successfully applying the 'handy approach' techniques, so it was suitable to take up the proposed research investigation on neonatal thermoneutral control, which Dr Ojuku frustrated its take-off at his hospital. The head of the unit, Dr Kumori, felt honoured to take part in the study and did not hesitate to conscript one of her resident doctors to allow him the opportunity to learn from the study. Dr Kumori was always available at all stages of the investigation, and with the assistance of her resident doctor, Dr Olutunde, the project went very smoothly. It was a beautiful study with very clear outcome. Many congratulations were showered on us by a lot of colleagues, nationally and internationally, on the outcome. I later commented on this study: 'Our hypothesis was positively confirmed, verified and finally published by *Paediatrics and International Child Health in 2015*. The question that kept ringing in my mind was whether some of our colleagues were there for the patients or for their personal egos. It was okay for anyone to be jealous of their own profession, but the colossal failure of Nigeria to achieve the neonatal component of the Millennium Development Goal (MDG4) target was because many paediatricians thought solutions must start and end with them. Unfortunately, modern medicine is inter-disciplinarily oriented and not just a 'one man show' venture'.

CMDs' club friendships

I enjoyed a very good institutional relationship with the CMDs' club and was often invited to their national conferences. I would particularly remember their Calabar conference during the time Professor Etawo was a chief medical director, and the Lagos conference during Professor Eugene's time as the CMD of one of the Federal Hospitals there. I made notable presentations to the delegates of these conferences, who mainly constituted the various CMDs of the federal government-owned tertiary health institutions. The conferences offered good blends of academic intellectualism mixed with business discussions for the progress of healthcare delivery in Nigeria.

My presence at all the conferences, mainly during the periods when Professor Kature and Professor Peter were chairmen of the club, was basically to deliver scientific papers on the numerous pieces of research I was carrying out to develop effective solutions to counter poor neonatal outcomes at the SCBUs of Nigerian hospitals. Many of the CMDs, especially those of them from the hospitals where I operated as a visiting consultant, looked forward to my presentations. They loved to hear me present the good progress their various hospitals were making in contrast to the sluggishness of their counterparts who had not deemed it necessary to join my growing research network and the campaign for drastic reduction of neonatal mortality across Nigeria. It was usually a delight to the collaborating CMDs to hear the results from me as I assessed the contributions of individual hospitals in the neonatal survival campaign. It motivated them to do more for the neonates. My presentations were often followed by comments and reactions from the various participating CMDs; other colleagues were usually challenged and motivated to initiate their own 'neonatal' projects as well.

It was usual for under-performing hospital CMDs to openly direct their anger towards me in the defence of the poor outcomes from their hospitals, as I experienced during one of the CMDs' club conferences. I flew to Nigeria in December of that year for the conference. Professor Kamuka chaired the session at Kano when I delivered my presentation on Nigeria neonatal progress one year before the end of MDG4. Ten CMDs signalled their desire for follow-up speeches or reactions based on the issues raised by my paper. Kamuka indicated interest to speak but would deny himself the slot, hence he would allow only eight speeches or reactions. Seven of the eight speeches were in agreement with the analyses showcased by my presentation, praising the positive impact of my outstanding consultancy at the various hospitals. However, one CMD was in opposition. She stated that I was a very difficult person who was full of discrimination. She said: 'This fellow does not deserve all the accolades colleagues have been showering on him because he was unnecessarily demanding whenever he was called upon to come and help at our hospital. Hippolite is high-minded, makes impossible demands and only goes where there is five-star hotel accommodation for him. In fact, he chooses where to go and snubs invitations from smaller hospitals he does not like, yet he is here telling us how much he loves Nigerian neonates'. There was open resentment and anger in her voice. She neither reported the state of her SCBU nor neonatal outcomes at her centre, or what she did with the periods of my consultancy at her hospital. She only concentrated on attacking my personality with baseless allegations. She failed to tell her colleagues that I had been visiting her SCBU to assist the centre until her later actions made me feel too uncomfortable to continue.

In my usual way, I refused to defend myself or counter-react to the bad report and accusations. I reasoned: 'I got such great comments from seven people out of eight – not too bad for me and the Nigerian neonates. If it was to be an exam, then that would yield an 'A-star' score'.

It was an open secret that I would unapologetically refuse to respond to the body language of some hospital staff or chief executives seeking any kind of gratification for whatever favour they felt I was receiving. This was one of those cases where I would quietly withdraw from a hospital when senior staff wanted to go 'outside the box' of saving the neonates. I might have wrongly perceived a couple of such advances from this CMD. I felt uncomfortable at this, especially as this related to a CMD of the opposite sex. I had had to resign my consultancy at the hospital and leave. I had to preserve my integrity and also circumvent the appearance of a scandal that would ruin my career for the Nigerian neonates.

When this woman was done speaking, spitting out her venom and expecting me to respond, everyone waited to hear what my defence would be. With a smile on my face, I folded up my laptop and said, 'Ladies and gentlemen, most respected CMDs, I thank you so very much for inviting me to make this presentation. Let us all remain strong and resolute for the neonates. This is a cause that none of us who understand would regret. Thank you again'. I began to walk back to my seat.

There were immediate reactions from the rest of the CMDs, from SCBUs where I had served, all refuting all the allegations and describing them as unfounded. Among the counter-voices was that of Professor Usman. Usman reacted: 'My honourable colleagues, I am at loss at our respected member's submission concerning Professor Hippolite. Madam may not be telling us everything…' – all laughed at this – 'Madam's hospital is located at the centre of a big city with beautiful houses, hotels and easy access roads, but mine is in a remote village in northern Nigeria, yet not even the rampaging of Boko Haram terrorists and bad access roads could stop Professor Hippolite from coming to us every six months. Madam, there may be another private dimension to your story.' There was another round of laughter. The CMDs' club was a fun group. Other members began to ask funny questions such as, 'Madam, did Hippolite 'toast' you?' Another colleague asked: 'Madam, it looks like this is really an unfinished 'something' with Hippolite. He is 'here-o', why not go privately and finish up with him?'

Each comment was hilarious and came with a round of laughter from the entertained ladies and gentlemen. Many other follow-up comments from delegates rendered the bad report pointless. In her attitude, this CMD did not seem to have the neonates as her priority. It was her indifferent attitude that had caused me to resign my consultancy at her hospital, so the neonates had continued to die there.

'What's in it for me?' The evil of civil servants

When a need arises, a job must be done. More often than not, external contractors were required to carry out jobs that ranged from supply of stationery to hard- and software-device maintenance. Various chains of command at the hospital come into play in the course of such jobs, from contractor interview to award of contract and from supervision to certification of completed project, and from finance/auditing to the cashier's desk for final payment. Government-paid civil servants in these chains of command were expected to treat the files professionally, and to move them to the next desk along the 'chain' until the contractor got his payment. Ideally, the contractor did not have to personally know every civil servant who would handle his/her file.

However, this was not so in my dreadful many years' experience of Nigeria. Every civil servant in the chain of command would insist on knowing what financial returns to expect from intending contractors – literally everyone, from management staff to accounting staff, from works department staff to internal auditors, and even the very head of the SCBU – at very few centres though. A contractor was expected to come over to make himself known to everyone 'relevant'. Contractors were always expected to 'see' these staff perhaps to negotiate the 'cuts' or, at least, befriend them. If this sycophantic friendship or bribe was not respected, the contractor would suffer terrible delays in the so-called government 'due process' for payment after job completion. There might even be premeditated outright disappearance of his contract file to frustrate his payment at the completion of the job.

My uncompromising non-compliance with these obnoxious illegal demands and bad practices was the number one reason why I was hated by many hospital staff and, hence, always a target for punishment. Some would say, 'Who does he think he is? Is he bigger than the other contractors who come to ensure that their files are being treated? We will work on his file when he is ready to come over here to settle us.'

As you have read, I was forced to learn my lesson from a lot of bad treatment I received from bribe-seeking civil servants at the very beginning of my career as a young engineer. Many of these shamelessly insatiable government workers were very senior officers who earned lots of money. Nevertheless, they were not much bothered about their poor patients provided their illegal gratifications and bribery proceeds were flowing in unhindered. As a young professional who was determined to follow the right path, I was often frightened to see how such highly-placed people would try to persuade me to abide by this norm. Some were not ashamed to communicate this verbally to me, while many used body language. These were unfortunate setbacks in my progress, both at the very beginning of my career and after my reputation and hard work had brought world-wide acolade. Twenty-five years of experience made no difference – the Nigerian civil servants got worse and worse, and more dishonest than ever. The corruption in Nigerian civil service circles was so malodorous that it respected no one, great or small. Much later, as a globally-respected professor at the prestigious Royal University, I still came face to face with shameless and audacious individuals who made the same approaches to me. Dishonesty was a canker that finished the Nigerian healthcare delivery services, sending countless patients to untimely graves. Sadly, the neonates were the worst hit.

I often resorted to threatening CMDs with immediate resignation from my services to the hospital when my payment was excessively delayed for no reasonable cause. Some CMDs would not pay attention to the complaints from me until they received such threats, perhaps to show that it had become imperative that an executive order was necessary to prevent contractual conflicts with me. These were the rare occasions when heads of indicted departments would try to avoid queries from the CMD, hence demand the immediate processing of my files for the payment of jobs done. One CMD told me that if he issued the 'matching order' prematurely, some hospital staff would label him a secret co-director of my fronting organisation (which was later renamed The Newlife Campaigns Limited); hence, my 'vested interest is to ensure quick payment,' he said. This claim was confirmed by a large number of decent hospital staff from the various tertiary hospitals across Nigeria. 'Why would you not happily accept the accusation of 'vested interest' and then explain what this means for you?' I asked. 'The immoral people's 'vested interest' is to steal money from the system, but your 'vested interest' is to avoid the death of your neonates by ensuring Hippolite is not frustrated. One is evil while the other is good. You should not allow the evil men to intimidate you. I would rather be bold and do the right thing for the poor patients,' I said.

Dr Kumori was a professional of decent character. She often sympathized with me when I decried the unnecessary hardships and frustrations that hampered my efforts to save the Nigerian babies. As a passionate paediatrician who had worked for many years alongside my research group, she understood how my contributions had been invaluable in recent neonatal success stories in Nigeria. However, she often found it difficult to understand it when I talked about my so-called 'administrative frustration'. I would explain that the hardest aspect of my job was neither the identification of chronic knowledge or technology gaps in neonatal practice, nor the synthesis of effective appropriate solutions, nor the delivery of these solutions to solve the actual problems. It was not even the very time-consuming clinical validation of these solutions.

The most difficult problem for me was not technical or clinical, but getting management staff to pay for jobs that had been delivered as agreed. I would pay no attention to these demands, no matter the language used, so the fight would normally end in my resignation.

Dr Kumori never understood, until it happened at her own hospital after her good CMD was succeeded by another one who was not so good. She got a note from the new CMD that my appointment had been terminated with immediate effect. This followed my earlier mail to the CMD vehemently criticising his deceptive promises, and stating my unpreparedness to accept double standard behaviours against me and the neonates. My withdrawal from the hospital generated debates across the various managers and staff of the administrative and accounts departments, some visibly expressing their happiness that I had been kicked out. Dr Kumori was shocked to hear many of these hospital staff openly attacking the SCBU and paediatrics staff, saying that they were the only people that Professor Hippolite shared gratification money with, and it never got to them. In shock, Dr Kumori complained: 'You guys surely did not know this 'Professor-o' if you thought he distributed money to anyone, anywhere. I am not only disappointed, I am ashamed, if this was the reason many of you ganged up against him without knowing that our own neonates would be the ones to suffer from his withdrawal. Clearly many of you don't realise that he is a top professor from a top international university, and he does not need us to remain who he proudly is'.

Dr Kumori sent her apologies to me on behalf of her co-staff at the hospital for my ill treatment after many years of benefiting from my services to the hospital.

Yanikis's professional protection

A situation I perceived as unnecessary protection of 'professional territory' from 'invaders' was a sad factor that added to the reason why Nigerian neonates died. Some Nigerian professionals rejected interdisciplinary collaboration as they tried to prove that they were the only authorities and hope for the survival of Nigerian neonates, but at the same time they rejected those who had been able to make a meaningful contribution. Hence, in the attempt to ward off the 'intruders,' they closed the inter-professional collaboration doors that could have helped in synthesising effective solutions to save the neonates.

Dr Yanikis had been trained at one of the best institutions in Australia and became a consultant perinatologist quite early in life. He quickly rose in academic rank and became a Professor of Perinatal Medicine in one of Nigeria's university teaching hospitals, the Uga University Hospital in Bendel State. Professor Yanikis was well respected amongst paediatricians in Nigeria. He was also very active in professional organisations and had the privilege of serving as a sponsored delegate in many child health conferences both within and outside Nigeria. Many other professors at the University of Uga respected Yanikis. He was so proud of himself – his academic and professional achievements, the respect and worship of colleagues he enjoyed and the fact that many saw him as their great leader and idol. This state of mind was not particularly good for Yanikis, as he began to let his pride take over. It was not too long before he started feeling and acting like a clinical mini-god, and the only 'champion' who had to be listened to. His hatred and resentment of some emerging names in his field of practice was not hidden as he castigated the perceived impacts they were making.

Yanikis and six other professional colleagues were on their way as sponsored delegates to a conference in Orlando, Florida. Their flight schedule from Abuja was routed via Glasgow airport, where they had a two-hour delay before boarding their flight to Orlando. This was a great time to chat about the challenges of neonatal healthcare in Nigeria. The very erudite Professor Aronge and Emeritus Professor Tobi were more senior professional colleagues in the team. Professor Aronge could not hide his excitement at all my achievements as I moved from one tertiary hospital to another, recovering broken-down neonatal incubators and enhancing the knowledge level of SCBU practitioners in paediatrics incubation techniques. The others in the team knew about my work and were all concurring with the good report from Professor Aronge.

'I really think our country needs more young, hard-working professionals like Hippolite, and must move fast to encourage our best brains such as this young man,' the professor continued with enthusiasm. 'This young chap lives in London, and who knows how long it will be before the white man keeps him too busy to have the time for his trips to help in Nigeria?'

Emeritus Professor Tobi nodded in agreement and added: 'When I first met the young man, I was the Chairman of the Board of Management of our hospital. We had to bring him along to turn around an almost hopeless situation in our SCBU. I doubted his ability initially, but as soon as I observed the passion in the young man, I did not hesitate any further before approving him for the job'.

'And how did he perform?' asked Aronge.

'Excellent, of course,' answered Tobi. 'My expectations for younger Nigerian professionals were reinvigorated when I got the report of successful completion of the job within two weeks of the contract award.'

Professor Yanikis looked lost as he stared from one person to another, listening as each person showered praises for what he/she had experienced or heard about the great jobs being done. 'Excuse me, but I don't get all this,' said Yanikis, with a surprised look on his face: 'This young man has a terrible record at my hospital. None of the engineers and technicians at my hospital has got a good thing to say about him. You guys seem to be talking about a different person'.

Professor Aronge interrupted: 'Yanikis, please can you shut up, as you don't seem to know the young engineer Hippolite. Is your comment out of tribal sentiments or have your engineers been denied their request for bribes, and so they decided to damage the young man's character? I know for sure that he has always been too decent for the bad fellows at our own Works Department. It is well known at my hospital that he openly refuses to give them money, so they hate him, but we still keep him to get our SCBU going.' There was silence for a while before the elderly Professor Tobi spoke: 'Yanikis, I must say that this is the first time I have heard a paediatrician make any negative report about Hippolite's performance'.

Back home in Nigeria after the Orlando conference, disaster struck. The SCBU of Uga University Hospital (UUH) had an unfortunate event where a neonate had died of severe burns from a hot water bottle spill. This was a huge problem for Professor Yanikis, being the Head of the Department of Paediatrics at the time. The management of the hospital needed an urgent answer for this. The disaster had been reported by the local newspaper and everyone was talking about how dangerous it was to seek medical intervention from such a callous hospital's SCBU. Lack of functional incubators was the major issue at stake, although the SCBU lacked other important devices for neonatal care as well. There was no functional incubator, so doctors would keep the hot water bottle inside a malfunctioning incubator, providing uncontrollable warming.

The embarrassment caused by this incident led to an urgent meeting of the top management committee of UUH, chaired by the CMD, Professor Tom. This meeting coincided with the period I was on my usual quarter-yearly medical mission trip in Nigeria. Professor Tom contacted me and arranged for me to present a proposal for the restoration of effective incubator care at his SCBU during the TMC meeting. Halfway into the session, I was called in to sit beside the CMD in the boardroom. He had notified all board members – and this included Professor Yanikis, who sat directly opposite the CMD – that I would be brought in to advise or make a presentation on possible options for restoring effective incubator interventions at the SCBU. The CMD introduced me and asked Professor Yanikis to briefly present the current status of the SCBU as related to the sad event that took place.

In his usual manner of speech, Yanikis sounded authoritative as he argued that his locally and internationally well-trained staff members were not overwhelmed by the problems at the SCBU: 'These are normal problems that are well known across all Nigerian SCBUs, not just here at UUH, and we are well able to tackle and resolve them'. Some sad members of the Board were itching to hear me speak on the matter, but none dared to challenge the powerful professor.

Professor Yanikis took a long time in his speech before the CMD signalled me to speak. I began: 'CMD, Director of Administration, Heads of Departments and others present, I thank you for this great honour of inviting me to provide input as you deliberate on how best to save the neonates in this part of the country. I am reasonably confident that this is a problem I can easily solve, and also take your doctors and nurses through training sessions that will definitely improve incubator care at your centre. I say this because I have tackled similar embarrassing situations in other hospitals. Some of you here, I am sure, are aware of this fact. The ugly situation of high neonatal mortality in Nigeria is due to both clinical and technical knowledge gaps that require urgent change or updating. So I will try to give you the clinical imperatives and later I will g…'

Before I could say the next word, Professor Yanikis interrupted: 'You do not have any qualifications to talk about clinical issues here. You are only a technician, what do you know about paediatrics and medicine?' He even went on to query my very presence in the meeting. What I thought to be a quick point of correction was turning out to be another lecture by the nerve-racking professor.

I sat down and allowed him to finish. His comments were insulting and intimidating, perhaps intended to utterly discredit me before the Board members. It was as though he hated the very air I was breathing. When he was done speaking, everyone waited for me to resume my speech, but I was quiet.

'We are waiting for you to continue,' the CMD said, looking

me in the face. 'Oh sir, are you? I didn't know,' I replied. 'The revered clinical professor can finish my speech, sorry'. Standing up and looking at the CMD in the eyes, I said: 'Thank you so much for inviting me, but I wish to be excused to go to other hospitals where I might be allowed to talk about clinical matters'. 'Oh no, you don't have to go,' said the CMD. But I headed for the exit door.

About seven months after this encounter, Professor Yanikis retired from service, having been the Head of the Paediatrics Department during these disastrous years. However, no one seemed to personally indict him for all the ugly things that happened under his watch. Another HOD took over from him, but the problems were not solved. Barely six months after his retirement, another disaster struck. This time, another neonate being monitored under an erratically uncontrollable radiant warmer was severely burnt and died as a result. The news quickly spread across Nigeria and was a big embarrassment to the Supreme Commander of the Federal Republic of Nigeria. Hence, a presidential order was released and the CMD and all his serving top management officials were dismissed from office. What a lucky fellow Professor Yanikis was. He successfully escaped the presidential disgrace that his colleagues had to face. His inaction, hatred and lack of respect for genuine passion were the reasons why neonates died at Uga centre.

How could he have escaped this, one would ask? It would have been only fair for some kind of disgraceful 'sacking' for Yanikis as others received. Neonates might have died, but their innocent blood would continue to cry out. If disgraceful sacking was God's intended punishment, did Yanikis really escape this? Do not jump to conclusions yet!

The year after this incident, Yanikis was appointed Nigerian Ambassador to the United Nations, and so became a big national figure. The name Yanikis became well-known even to common people in the marketplace, well beyond medical circles. Yanikis celebrated this with his friends. He felt invincible, but God and the lost neonates had not forgotten what he had done. He happily relocated to New York, USA, as the head of Nigerian diplomatic mission. In his new job and position, 'His Excellency, Ambassador the Professor Yanikis,' remained as highly prejudiced as ever. Then, at the very peak of Ambassador Yanikis's popularity, disaster struck. A well-publicised scandalous incident within government circles sadly indicted him, and the Nigerian Supreme Commander ordered his immediate recall for interrogation. Yanikis's poor judgements had finally landed him in trouble on the big stage. There was no hiding away or arrogant defence. The Supreme Commander had no choice other than to issue orders for his immediate dismissal. In a national broadcast of the presidential orders on the case, the highly respected and erudite scholar was shamed. It was a national humiliation. It might have been a coincidence, but any good done for the neonates would never been forgotten by posterity; so also was the evil done to these poor innocent humans. It did not matter if the evil was done by directly killing the neonates or indirectly, by stopping effective moves that could have saved them.

Neonatal blood money – mismanagement impunity

'If you cannot beat them, join them'. This has always been a common Nigerian saying. Another saying similar to this was:

'If you cannot beat them, let them'. I often commented: 'I think these sayings should be for the coward. For me, if I cannot beat them, I change my strategies and keep trying until I do beat them.' Sometimes there is wisdom in keeping quiet, provided the quietness is a strategy to beat evil. Keeping quiet was not necessarily a mark of being humble; in fact, most of the time, it was being cowardly. If a man felt he was good enough to fight the evil people in the rank and file of Nigerian politicians, if he was also good enough to fight the 'pen robber' among Nigerian civil servants, if after several attempts he failed to defeat these evils within the establishments where he worked, then what should he do? Many Nigerians would think that their failed efforts to stop evil should be enough justification to go for their own 'piece of the national cake' by releasing the hibernating devil in their own lives. However, it is rather foolish for someone to transform into a demon after a failed attempt to stop a Lucifer. His previous good acts would be forgotten, and all that would be remembered would be his later evil.

I was resolute in my ways; however, I was occasionally outsmarted by some evil people. Nonetheless, rather than joining them, I got even tougher in my relationships with them. My song of saving the neonates would always sound sympathetic and humanitarian to genuine people. At the same time it was easily used as a front by some heartless health workers to attract funds they would afterwards divert into their private pockets. They premeditated the cover-up that would follow, and then implemented their ever-effective looting games – all for the 'blood money' of the dying neonates and other patients dying from other tragic diseases.

Professor Obamawa, a renowned pathologist, was once the Chief Medical Director of a tertiary hospital. Obamawa had trained at one of London's prestigious hospitals during his earlier years of medical practice. He was passionate about neonates and could not stand to see their young lives wasted. When he assumed office as CMD he was immediately confronted with the frustration of the high neonatal mortality rate, blamed largely on lack of functional incubators. This was during the early days of my career, when my neonatal incubator skills were only known to about four Nigerian tertiary hospitals. Professor Obamawa heard about me and decided to give me a trial, though he was not too sure what I could do.

I arrived and after a couple of days, I succeeded in providing the needed solution, restoring a number of the incubators to their functional capacities. Professor Obamawa was delighted with me, and our professional friendship continued all through the years of Obamawa's tenure. Professor Obamawa's kindness and true passion for the neonates endeared him to me; he occupied such a place of high regard in my heart that the long separation whilst I studied in London could not wipe this out. He loved my hard work for making sure that the special care baby unit of his hospital remained one of the great successes of his administration all through his time in office.

Many years later, I had become a consultant orthopaedics biomechanist at the Royal University, and Obamawa was delighted to contact me during one of his visits to the UK. I arranged a lunch meeting at a luxury London restaurant near Hyde Park. Obamawa was fascinated by how much knowledge I had acquired in modern keyhole surgical interventions. He said: 'Hippolite, I cannot wait to bring you to Nigeria to speak in one of our conferences. I often get lost in international conferences when western specialists begin to display this kind of high skill in mathematical orthopaedics and image analysis in their presentations. I often try to imagine Nigeria getting to this stage, but here you are today at the cutting edge of this class of orthopaedic biomechanics.'

Professor Obamawa was often referred to as 'the father of skilful practice' in Nigeria and was well-respected among doctors. He wanted his Nigerian colleagues to be inspired by my scientific achievements, so he worked furiously to get me invited as a guest speaker at the Nigerian Medical Society conference in Ekulobia in 2007.

My presentation on 'engineering the human joints' expounded on my development of predictive tools for planning keyhole surgery of the glenohumeral joint of the upper limb. The presentation was like a scientific magical movie to many participants, as three-dimensional simulation of the motions of articulating shoulder bones was new at the time. One particular paediatrician, Dr Fatai, sat in awe as I made my presentation. Delighted with the talk, he stated: 'I am pleased that at last, a Nigerian professional can stand on our local podium to display the same kind of presentation we often watch on cable television from developed countries'. He came forward after the session and congratulated me for my speech whilst Professor Obamawa, as the brain behind my invitation, looked on with pride.

Professor Obamawa introduced Dr Fatai as the Chief Medical Director of Otoko University Hospital, telling him, 'Hippolite is a man of many parts. He can also solve your neonatal incubator problems, no matter how bad your situation might be.'

'Really,' said Dr Fatai. 'In that case Doctor Hippolite, would you like to come to my hospital without delay, please? I have got real problems with lack of functional incubators at the moment'.

I visited the OUH and for the two years that followed, I established a regular consultancy visit to the hospital's SCBU. My activities at the hospital became a great success, which the CMD was always happy to cite in his list of achievements as the CMD of the hospital. Unfortunately, Dr Fatai faced a lot of trouble with some people in the political class that managed the Ministry of Health. The politicians influenced appointments of chief executives of government-owned facilities such as Otoko University Hospital. Many politicians of the ruling party were jobless and were known for hanging around the chief executives of government establishments asking for contracts from them, and threatening to get them sacked if they didn't comply. It was a regular thing at the OUH, and the chairman of the ruling party was frequently seen patrolling the walkways of the hospital. Very often he would try to compel the CMD to allow him to influence and inflate contract awards and use other methods to divert public funds into his private pocket, as claimed by this CMD. The CMD's fight against this was endless as the politicians never gave up. Dr Fatai would often say to me, 'I am really getting tired of these people. How could they secretly come here and take away all the money meant for running the hospital, and when there is poor hospital outcome owing to lack of funds, they turn around and blame me?'

Dr Fatai refused the demands as often as he could. However, this infuriated them all the more, so they fabricated a lie against him and quietly sacked him from office, replacing him with another person who shared their mind-set. During the years I visited the hospital as a consultant, my friendship with the sacked CMD grew so strong that we were happy to keep in touch with each other afterwards.

This CMD's experience was a classical story of Nigerian political victimisation. Dr Fatai's virtue paid him back, as four years later the Federal Government, under a new president, offered him an appointment as the Executive Secretary of the Federal Ministry of Health. He now became a superintending executive at the federal level. In a sense, he became the boss of those who had been his recent bosses. Dr Fatai's tenure would only last ten months, so he had no time to waste in making an impact.

For or against the neonates?

After about a month in office, Dr Fatai, as the new Executive Secretary (Superintendent) of the health ministry, invited me for a discussion in his new office following my request for a meeting. I planned the date to coincide with the period of my regular medical mission trip to Nigeria. I flew in from London and stayed a while at Abuja to be able to keep the appointment. I was surprised when I showed up at the appointed time only to be told that Dr Fatai, the Superintendent, would not be able to see me because he was not there. His secretary gave me the option of coming back the next day. Superintendents were often called upon for one errand or another outside their official scheduled daily appointments by the Honorable Minister of Health.

The meeting was rescheduled three times. I was displeased because of all my time being wasted, but, I did not easily give up since I believed I had one thing in common with Dr Fatai – a passion for neonatal survival. I had no doubt we were going to have a good meeting, but never knew the format this would take. It was not clear if Dr Fatai was going to invite some senior Ministry of Health (MoH) staff to listen to me talk about what I had been doing so well in Nigeria. The Superintendent did not need to be convinced of the authenticity or efficacy of my RIT incubator systems, but perhaps he was interested in getting information on how I intended to tweak operations to coordinate a new federal project to assist the neonates through the nation-wide coverage of his ministry.

I prepared a PowerPoint presentation, not knowing the form the meeting would take. I also ensured that my pocket-size multimedia projector was in my bag, just in case it came in handy. I arrived in good time and waited in the visitors' seating area for over five hours until about eight o'clock in the night when a young staff member of the MoH walked in with a piece of paper in his hand. He was dressed in a neat pink shirt and black velvet trouser with a tie to match. He looked around all the men and a woman seated: 'Who is Doctor Hippolite?' he asked. I raised my hand. 'Can you follow me, please?' he said.

The young man led me to the Superintendent's secretary. There was another chair to sit upon for ten more minutes before the security signal on the large metal framed door flashed green with accompanying chime. 'Okay, Doctor, you can go in,' said the secretary as he reached out and opened the door for me.

Across an 'island' seating area in an open space with a massive office desk sat the face I had known for over four years. The smile beaming from his face was one of victory as if to say: 'Can you see me now? I have got the last laugh now after the injustices I suffered as the head of the tertiary hospital where you knew me.' There was no one else in the office.

I knew how much Dr Fatai had suffered at the hands of his bosses because he would not accept their evil ways. I wished that everyone who suffered injustice in the Nigerian health sector, especially for the sake of the neonates, could one day be so promoted and honoured. Dr Fatai deserved the elevation for all he had endured fighting for the patients in the city of Otoko.

A quick look around the intimidating huge office made me feel a bit nervous. Later I found it difficult to understand why I had been so nervous. Although the Superintendent was an old friend, this was the first time I had been in the office of a national superintendent. It was already late in the night and I was conscious of the fact that I had left about five other people in the waiting area. I decided not to waste any time but to go straight to the discussion – a typical British common sense.

Dr Fatai remained seated whilst I walked up to greet him. 'Good evening, Honourable Superintendent,' I said, stretching out my hand. Dr Fatai accepted the handshake, still smiling. 'You are welcome engineer, please sit down,' he responded. 'It's been a long time.' He looked down, reading through a document in his hand. This was the proposal I had submitted many weeks earlier requesting this meeting. 'Is he just reading it for the first time or trying to remember the high points in the write-up?' I was wondering.

There was a brief silence, so to break it I brought out my mini laptop computer in the attempt to begin my speech. The Superintendent had known me too well and noticing my nervous state of mind, he said: 'Engineer, relax; I know what you are capable of doing. I have an idea of how we shall go about this.' He lifted up the document in his hand. 'This is your proposal; I will tell you what we are going to do to assist the Nigerian neonates. I know this is your passion and it is my desire to help too'.

I regained my composure and waited for the superintendent to finish his reading. He took his green pen and wrote instructions on the paper, looked up and said: 'I am passing this on to one of our directors in the ministry to work with you to ensure this project is carried out.'

In the document, I had made proposals based on my wide experience of neonatal shortcomings across Nigeria. I had appealed to the Ministry to step up action for the provision of sustainable incubators for the teeming population of tiny babies being born across Nigeria. The document cited the great exploits of my Recycled Incubator Technology (RIT) and how these techniques had been used to provide adequate incubator intervention in SCBUs around Nigeria. A line in the document read, 'All of us in the ranks and levels of neonatal special care in this country cannot deny the fact that high neonatal mortality is a problem we can solve with this effective technique if only we can eschew dishonesty to genuinely move to save the Nigerian neonate.'

The Superintendent knew all about my previous cynicism towards the insincerity of Federal Ministry of Health (FMoH) workers. During the early days of our friendship, we discussed how we detested the FMoH staff, their greed and inappropriate behavious. This was long before Dr Fatai got the elevated job of Federal Superintendent. Whenever I was on my routine consultancy visit to Dr Fatai's department at his former place of work, we related very well and spent evenings together. We passionately discussed the ills of Nigeria's healthcare system and the incompetence of some civil servants in the state and federal ministries of health. We both wished someone reasonable would one day be in charge of these ministries and change things. Neither of the two 'great minds' ever suspected that within a few years, Dr Fatai himself could secure the executive position of the very office we blamed.

I was very happy for Dr Fatai when the news of his appointment was made public. I did not hesitate to congratulate my old friend through an email, and later, a telephone call. I must balance my relationship with Dr Fatai in the most appropriate manner this time. This was necessary in order to distinguish myself from the teeming population of sycophants crowding around the new superintendent. Part of my message to Dr Fatai read: 'I rejoiced when I heard of your appointment but must remind you of our numerous discussions on the state of healthcare delivery systems in Nigeria. I am so happy for you but do regret one thing only – you have been appointed into the most difficult ministry in Nigeria. I promise to keep praying for you but watch your back! I hope my friend can finish doing this work and still remain stainless…'

I remained quiet for some time as I sat across from the Superintendent imagining how I could work with a FMoH director, and looking him in the eye I said: 'Honourable Superintendent, you know as well as I do that many of these civil servants are not here for the dying poor Nigerian patients but for their own pockets. Can we not find an alternative method of effectively using your short term in this office to make a huge impact across the nation in neonatal survival without involving these gullible people who really never cared about the needs of the neonates? I am afraid, but my gut feeling tells me that once these people are brought into the implementation of this idea they may only hatch a plan to use it for fund embezzlement, and they will eventually kill the idea.'

'Oh not so, trust me Hippolite, I am assigning the implementation to someone who will never disappoint the neonates, trust me,' he replied.

'Is he or she a director in this ministry?' I asked with a surprise look at the Superintendent.

'Yes, he is the Director of Local Medicine in the ministry. He is Dr Onwukwuo, a very trustworthy person. I will personally instruct him to ensure that this project is successfully executed,' said the Superintendent.

As two old friends we had a brief catch-up about other personal subjects, and I thanked him again for inviting me and left. The file was passed on to Dr Onwukwuo the next day. He extracted my local and UK phone numbers from the proposal document he had received and gave me a call to notify me that he had been detailed by the Superintendent to supervise my proposed neonatal project.

Dr Onwukwuo swiftly invited me to another meeting where he assembled a panel of 12 senior staff of the FMoH, including some other junior directors, to listen to the presentation of my ideas, and to discuss the possible strategies for the implementation of the project. Onwukwuo welcomed me and all the members to the round-table discussion, announcing that I would make a presentation on High Neonatal Mortality Rate in Nigeria and what could be done to drastically lower this.

He invited each person to introduce him/herself before the presentation began. I keenly looked at the faces of each panel member as they introduced themselves. I looked each of them in the eye as if to say: 'Tell me, are you here for your pocket or for the neonates?' I had my doubts about these people but it was not time to reject them before testing their intentions.

I put my presentation setup together and thanked everyone in the room for the opportunity to talk about the most important issue in my heart. I paused and once again looked directly into the eyes of everyone seated at the conference table, whilst nodding, a gesture that everyone noticed.

'I can fully recognise only one person here and she might know me through her former university professor, who is my very good friend. So, apart from Dr Margaret, has anyone here heard about me or my work amongst the Nigerian SCBUs before my letter to the FMoH?' I asked.

Three people signalled 'yes', so I began my presentation without telling them why I had asked that question. The success stories of the RIT approach to incubator restoration was demonstrated as part of my talk. During question time, a number of the participants described the information and data presented about the various states of the SCBUs across the country as very educative. I carefully answered all questions from the FMoH staff. I was emphatic as I declared: 'funding is necessary to save our neonates; however, this is not the most important factor for success. If we really want to save these babies, then the most important factor would be 'thinking'.

So you have got to put on your thinking caps. Many Nigerian professionals and so-called intellectuals are too busy chasing irrelevant superficial factors other than thinking how to articulate proper solutions. People are fond of blaming their failures on lack of money; yet when the money is provided, they mismanage it without solving the problem. Nigerians spend 80% of the time discussing and chasing funds but less than 20% of the time in thinking to generate and synthesise the right ideas. I declare that 80% thinking time will achieve far better successes even with only 20% of fund-raising time. We can only save the neonates by changing our current strategies as these have failed and continued to fail.'

I concluded with this challenge: 'I have a real problem here. I don't want to pre-empt anyone's score for this project, but I need everyone here to work hard enough to prove my cynicism wrong. I have this awful belief that civil servants at the FMoH are primarily here to fill their pockets rather than to work to save the dying patients. As we plan to work together, you have two challenges from me: one, to prove my cynical attitude wrong and hence two, to save the neonates.'

Dr Onwukwuo gave a vote of thanks to me, promising that the proposal was a great project that would never fail. He rescheduled another meeting for the next day to draw up the strategy for project implementation. I was again present to provide guiding information.

Dr Onwukwuo and his team needed me to agree on a course of action, and to co-sign the working document for the Federal Superintendent to approve the release of implementation funds. He created another three-man team and gave them a copy of my proposals with the instruction to produce a draft working document for discussion during the meeting. This was the document to be agreed upon, once tweaked for the Superintendent's approval.

I was full of doubts when I went through the produced document. The project was divided into three phases: (1) Travelling round all federal tertiary hospitals in the country to ascertain the total number of functional incubators at each SCBU – this was to be completed within the first two months; (2) Establishing regional stations where these incubators would be brought for examination and recycling – to be completed within the second two months; (3) the recycling of the assembled incubator systems, to commence by the sixth month. I frowned at this and wondered how two whole months was allocated for travelling round the country in teams of two senior staff that would spend two days at each SCBU location, only to ascertain the total number of functional incubators – information that could easily be obtained by telephone calls within two days. I told the directors that the document did not look real or reflect the urgency that the project implied.

Dr Onwukwuo tried to persuade me that doing this in phases as suggested would help to keep the project in motion as the funding was not fully available for the entire work. I hesitated but later agreed to sign the document after my old friend, Dr Fatai, vouched again for Dr Onwukwuo's ability to ensure project fulfilment. The Superintendent did not delay his approval for releasing the funds as soon as the working document was passed to him. I left for the UK after one week.

However, I discovered that five weeks after the Superintendent's approval to release funds, no SCBU in the country had been visited for this purpose. The reason I received upon enquiry was that no money had been found in any of the appropriate funding accounts to implement the approved fund. I called Dr Onwukwuo in frustration to object to this unnecessary delay, demanding again: 'why can't we override this visitation stage by simply making telephone calls to the SCBUs to gather this information? We shall save huge costs on transportation, feeding and hotel bills for two senior FMoH staff travelling outside Abuja city.'

Dr Onwukwuo would not give in but insisted on delaying the start of the project until money had been given to him to initiate the travelling. I patiently waited until the beginning of the 8th week. I called Dr Onwukwuo again and was told that some money had been found and released from the accounts termed 'Hospital Services' of the ministry; hence, the commencement of the SCBU visits would be in another two weeks.

My frustration continued to mount after nearly five months from the approval date, when I discovered that only the Kamalu Tertiary Hospital had been visited out of over 25 federal tertiary hospitals scheduled. My doubts heightened as I began to feel used by these enemies of the Nigerian neonate. This was compounded by the fact that Dr Fatai's tenure as the Superintendent would end in slightly more than three months. I sought to know the reason why Dr Onwukwuo and his colleagues were so slow to complete their so-called phase 1 of the project, despite the fact that the travel funding cost had been fully spent. I decided to call Dr Margaret for answers since I believed that she might not hide the truth from me.

Dr Margaret explained that money had been released but 'Oga,' meaning Dr Onwukwuo, had chosen to appoint only four people to make up the two groups that would visit all the

SCBUs. She continued: 'I am one of the four, however, money is given to us on a trip-by-trip basis – that is, money is put in our account to travel whenever Oga deems fit to dispatch us.'

This explained who the 'monster' was. Six and half months of the project timeline had passed but only two hospital SCBUs had been visited. The enthusiasm demonstrated by all the people who had attended the earlier seminar had evaporated. None of them called me for updates any more. All the team members began to behave as if the project was already over. It looked as if they had obtained all they were looking for. The Superintendent himself was hardly taking my calls when I tried to reach him in the ensuing frustration. It was becoming obvious that this was another classical scam of the FMoH staff; this time led by Dr Onwukwuo – a doctor, a man, a father and perhaps a grandfather.

I did not bother to call anyone again for another six weeks, as it was only two months to the end of Dr Fatai's tenure in office. I had made up my mind that I had been duped, and I was no longer prepared to continue with the project, no matter what excuses and lies Dr Fatai or Dr Onwukwuo told.

Shortly after this, I was one week into my quarterly medical mission trip in Nigeria. I was in Lagos executing my consulting slot for one of the SCBUs of the Oregun Federal Teaching Hospital. I woke up that very morning feeling completely useless in the hands of the 'caterpillars' at the FMoH. My thoughts ran through all my personal expenditure, attending several meetings and flight costs from London and within Nigeria – expenses I gladly incurred for the sake of the neonates. I thought about the babies whose deaths I had witnessed in the SCBU the previous day, and how many of these died of preventable causes. I thought of the fat-looking FMoH men whose eyes I had stared into during my presentation eight months earlier at Abuja. I thought of how honest-looking Dr Onwukwuo was, but how he had turned out to be another 'anaconda' that ate up neonates. The anger was welling up in my heart; so I decided to make my very last phone call to Dr Onwukwuo. I was not prepared to be Mr Nice Guy anymore. The rage in my heart had removed the lamb and brought in the lion.

I moved into a quiet room, pulled out my mobile phone and dialled Dr Onwukwuo's number. 'Poom-poom, poom-poom... 'If you want this tone for fifty naira, then press one',' his phone responded, and then began to recite Psalm 23 – 'The Lord is my Shepherd, I shall not want ...' I was amused at how deceitfully religious this man was, wondering if he would pick up his phone before I got to the last word of Psalm 23. Nigerians love to substitute the standard ringtone with their favourite music or political or religious messages. Mobile phone providers normally offer this service at one-off cost of 50 naira only.

'Hello,' answered Dr Onwukwuo.

'Hi Dr Onwukwuo, this is Hippolite - Dr Amadi,' I replied.

'It appears you are in the country. Are you planning to come and see us in Abuja?' asked Dr Onwukwuo.

'I only visit people who care about the poor Nigerian neonates. Have you got any positive information on the progress of my project, as that is the only thing that can bring me to Abuja?' I replied.

'I'm afraid not, the Ministry still doesn't have money to progress on the project and...' Dr Onwukwuo was beginning his usual cock and bull story, but I interrupted him: 'Oga, please keep your endless empty stories to yourself, because I have heard enough of your lies. You knew what you wanted to do right from the very inception of this project, and I guess you have already achieved it. It was really never your plan to do anything for the neonates. You guys at the FMoH have done what you know how to do best – to dupe dying Nigerian patients. When will you all be satisfied with the blood money you are using to fill your pockets? When shall…'

At that point, 'poom-poom-poom,' the line went off, but I would not give up. I redialled Dr Onwukwuo, not expecting that he would take the call, but he did, and I continued: 'You collected the budget money to complete your so-called phase 1 of the project but in the last eight months, you and your colleagues visited only two hospitals. Who are you continuing to deceive? Never mind, I will not accept any more collaboration with you. You are evil – the very enemy of the neonates. Many of them are dying due to your wickedness. I donate their corpses to you. I hope you will be happy to fry them and eat them – no point burying them. You should be ashamed of yourself.'

Having finished pouring out my heart, I paused. I never imagined that the dreaded Dr Onwukwuo would patiently absorb this angry outburst. He responded: 'I don't normally let people talk to me the way you have done this morning. You…' But before he could say the next word, I interrupted: 'Then you should have cut me off'.

'Oh yes, I could have done that, but for my respect for the honourable Superintendent as I know he is your very good friend,' he responded.

My anger was beginning to rise again: 'I have finished with you, Dr Onwukwuo. I must let you continue your game without me, so I can go and find possible help for the poor neonates elsewhere'. I hung up and quickly sent an email to my friend, Dr Fatai, regretting all the mess I had suffered at the hands of Dr Onwukwuo and his insatiable desire for dirty cash.

CHAPTER 11

HOW MDG(4) WAS DOOMED TO FAIL

✦✦✦✦✦✦✦

The United Nations' Millennium Development Goals (MDG) were a carefully-crafted developmental plan by the global body to accelerate the improvement of all global communities towards better environments, good health and prosperous economies. The 25 years of MDG have come and gone, having been launched in 1990. Wise countries, societies and agencies have assessed their successes and failures, re-strategizing to find possible ways of sustaining the various successes the MDGs achieved.

The huge projects executed around the world during the

MDG era required huge funding. Hence, the period saw all kinds of fund-raising and fund-consuming agencies and campaigns. This was necessary as the projects could not be realised without the funds. However, 'funds without effective thinking will never realise any projects'. This saying could be better understood now that societies are counting their failures and financial wastage. It was more painful for situations where huge amounts of money went into operators' pockets over the entire 25 years without a clear realisation of the target, or even significant progress towards it. In such cases, it would be a crime against humanity to ignore a 'review' of the colossal failure in concerned societies or countries such as Nigeria, where there was no 'significant' progress towards the reduction in mortality of neonates. We might debate what constitutes failure and success, but this is simple to resolve. There was a target, right? Failure to achieve this target within the provided quarter of a century constituted a failure, period! As should be expected of modern-day public servants, the individuals and committees that captained or served the government and academia during this period of capital failure should recognise their shame, bury their faces and resign in disgrace. Yet in Nigeria, they were still being seen moving around with their empty philosophies. Many individuals and organisations enriched themselves through the various programmes regardless of the apparent lack of impact being made with such methods in the reduction of neonatal mortality, for example. They were only after the money they realised through these hoax programmes, and never bothered if the neonates were really surviving commensurately with the amount of money being spent.

Nigerian academia, with its countless incompetent professors, lacked the ingenuity to create new ideas or investigate the imported ones for proper tweaking. They never researched to scientifically question the mode of application or the use of all kinds of foreign ideas being dumped on Nigeria. Instead, what mattered most to these individuals was juicy foreign and local collaboration money which oiled their unlimited desire to mismanage public funds. These people hid behind so-called government policies and focused on their personal shares of diverted funds instead of measuring impacts by real predictive research, articulating the 'killer factors' and synthesising the best applications that would guarantee the survival of Nigeria neonates.

One of the major targets of the MDG in Nigeria, dubbed MDG(4), was the reduction of the mortality rate of children under five years of age (U5) by a factor of 67% within the said 25-year period. The dual targets of reduction of maternal and child mortality became hot topics within the Nigerian health sector. Civil servants in the ministries of health, pharmaceuticals and the tertiary hospitals spoke compassionately about high rates of mortality during the day, but at night they perfected their endless schemes of siphoning all available funds into their own pockets. Huge sums of money – in the order of hundreds of millions of US dollars – through federal government appropriations, state government allocations and foreign government donations were squandered and covered up with fictitious documents and made-up scientific data. Hence the MDG4 would go down in history as the most atrocious wickedness of Nigeria against her own newly-born babies, infants and little children.

For the infants (one month to 12 months old) and older U5s, some relative reduction of mortality could be measured. This was largely attributed to imported vaccines for immunization of infants that survived the deadly neonatal period of life. However for the neonates (babies within the first 28 days of life), the imported ideas were unsuccessful, and the Nigerian scientific community did not have the balls to innovate own functional solutions. Hence, no significant progress could be measured towards reduction of neonatal mortality. It was a colossal failure and a national shame by all standards.

By the end of 2015, the world had technically left Nigeria behind to move on because the United Nations launched her Sustainable Development Goals (SDG) Programmes to replace the MDG. The SDG goal 3.2 (SDG3.2) target was to 'end preventable deaths of newborns and under-five children by the year 2030'. According to the 2015 demographic indicators published by UNICEF, Nigeria succeeded in reducing U5 mortality rate by only 42% against the expected target of 67%. Majority of the lives saved were from the older categories of the U5 children as the neonates accounted for most of the remaining 25% of the target. As Nigeria is still miles away from the erstwhile MDG4 target, should we join the rest of the world going into the SDG3.2 era without first analysing and understanding why our MDG4 was a failure? In this review, a journey could be taken in retrospect through the years to assess what could be seen as the failure factors without which the MDG4 success could have been guaranteed.

I stepped into the Nigerian scene of the MDG4 era in 1996, so I became actively involved during the last fifteen years of the 25-year race. The factors that contributed to the colossal

Nigerian failure of MDG(4) could hence be mirrored through my observations.

A vision born, a target set

In the beginning, a clear need was identified regarding the high death rate of children under five. Existing academic work within the Nigerian practice provided enough evidence for this need. By the assessment of prevailing statistics, large numbers of children would die from preventable causes before the age of five. The MDG call by the United Nations to her member countries was pleasing to Nigeria; hence, Nigeria joined the race to reduce the U5 mortality rate by two-thirds by the year 2015. The job would have been 'all hands on deck' for the various national governments in policy formulations as UN agencies/organisations released guidelines via resource and information sharing across member nations.

A good number of countries understood the need and were very serious about this, unlike Nigeria. Factors contributing to high neonatal mortality rate (NNMR) must be discovered and solutions synthesised against these. The various factors perceived to be contributing to this problem were being identified and published across the world, including Nigeria. Some countries funded their universities to research and synthesise own solutions, but Nigeria, in her scientific laziness, only waited to apply whatever solutions other countries developed. A success-oriented project technique would require a careful assessment of the subject problem to determine the specifics of its enhancement, perhaps based on race, demography, climate and culture, so as to devise an adequate solution that could eradicate or mitigate this.

The World Health Organisation, UNICEF and other global organisations could roll out programmes of suggested solutions based on findings from various countries; however, it was left for the other adopting nations to copy these in such a sensible manner as to guarantee anticipated results in their own settings. The required tweaking was the duty of the incountry government policy makers, hospitals and research institutions. Policies should however not be set arbitrarily but based on scientifically validated investigations hinging on other influencing local factors – climatic, cultural, ethnic and social dynamics, as these might vary from the country of origin of the very solutions or ideas being copied. Hence, any solution that was very sensitive to culture and climate, for example, was susceptible to failure if these dimensions were not knowledgeably tweaked.

Did Nigerian academic and healthcare professors get this aspect of the scientific debate right? Certainly not! Countries that implemented ideas 'hook, line and sinker' without local factor-based justification may have lacked the self-drive for independent research or lacked confidence in the ability of their local medical academics to generate trustworthy data. Therefore, Nigerian academia was a major contributor to the failure of MDG4. This brings to the fore the unavoidable role that should have been played by academia through research, based on true quest for academic knowledge and not illicit drives to amass financial wealth through shoddy deals with FMoH 'caterpillars' who devoured money out of sheer greed.

Nigeria neglected the fundamental key to technological

growth and hence squandered the 25 years set aside to restore the hopes of several millions of Nigerian neonates who died of preventable causes. Government, industry and academia (GIA), the tripod of advancement of technology, must work with equal mutual respect if any country desires to independently progress in the provision of optimal technologies to address her needs, including healthcare.

It was the duty of those in power to use the machinery of checks and balances to ensure that time and money being spent was effectively addressing the factors that would keep the neonatal survival target on track. Programmes that were not producing commensurate results should have been recalled for review, rethink or outright removal. The recalled funds from discontinued programmes should have been redirected to other better, more effective and result-oriented programmes. The Nigerian government functionaries were really not after quality results, or channelling funds in the direction of solutions that could save more neonates. No, good results were not their private or collective agenda. Typically, any programme that enabled diversion of public funds into their personal pockets had their blessing. Hence, they were ever ready to collaborate with any willing foreign or local agencies to get such monies 'spent,' whether or not the programme provided good healthcare values for the amount being spent. These unethical practices were well known, but no one challenged them. Senior government officials turned a blind eye. This bunch of educated offenders against the neonates forgot that expenditure without commensurate success would amount to failure. These government functionaries, including federal ministers of health, state commissioners of health, senior civil servants of the ministries of health, professors and senior academics of the tertiary hospitals, legislators, state governors and presidents – who were all parts of the formulation of the policies and financial cover-ups of the failed era – refused to question the dangerous 'expenditure without good results'. I collectively call them the destroyers, the neonatal murderers or the 'caterpillars' of the failed era. They kept quiet because their individual private pockets were taken care of at the detriment of the blood of millions of Nigerian newborns.

The caterpillars and their foreign masters

It could be counterproductive for countries to live in isolation, outside the committee of other nations and global bodies such as the WHO, World Bank, UNICEF etc, in their pursuit of a successful MDG era. However, every country was fully responsible for her actions and inactions. The global bodies were only there in advisory roles and for information dissemination across the wider world. Every seemingly effective approach announced by any country, research institution or organisation ought to have been strictly scrutinised and reassessed against Nigeria's social, cultural and climatic factors before adoption or adaption and eventual commitment of our resources. The greedy 'caterpillars' accepted virtually every proposal from the white man through the so-called 'donor countries', who only impoverished Nigeria by dangling 'units' in her face with one hand whilst stealing 'hundreds' from her with the other. It required self-confidence, smartness and unselfishness to spot the 'hidden agenda'. The caterpillars lacked these virtues, so the policies, methods and approaches were acceptable to them provided they came from the light-skinned foreigner. The inferiority complex and slavish mentality of these caterpillars sank the Nigerian neonate.

Foreign nations worked hard and developed their culturally and climatically compliant technologies to resolve issues of child health in their countries. Their research institutions were adequately funded and tasked just to produce the technologies that would combat their problems. They created solutions, published their findings, wrote books and then moved on to optimize the technologies. Conversely, the caterpillars never challenged academia, never cared about local technologies or development of any perceived discoveries. They were all perfect in identifying the latest technologies by foreign nations, and sold the entire country by the importation of every relevant and irrelevant technology irrespective of its compatibility with our climate and culture. They reduced Nigeria to one of the most technologically lazy countries in the world, importing toothpicks, rice, palm oil, petrol and 'keke-napepe' amongst other ludicrous agricultural and technological products.

The caterpillars allowed their slavish mentality to rob them of sensible questions that could have challenged the white lies that were controlling and empowering Nigeria's laziness to think and create. Skin-to-skin mother care technique, otherwise called kangaroo mother care (KMC), was a low-cost method of keeping babies warm in the absence of a technologically-controlled thermal environment. The technique could easily become ineffective in cases of extreme prematurity, that is, when a neonate's birthweight is below 1000g. Neonatal incubator technology was expensive to acquire, being imported, but the design and production of this technology could not be classified as rocket science. Nigeria could possibly have developed its own climate-compliant incubator models through concerted research. Such a brand could have been mass produced to support Nigeria's vast neonatal thermal need. Without considering the lack of sustainable results in these foreign models, the caterpillars continued importation of these devices, sadly in inadequate quantities. The few incubators that were provided were poorly maintained. These would be overused for a while without adequate maintenance and would soon pack up. The foreign engineers were not available to fix the broken-down systems. The spare parts supply chains were poorly established, but this never bothered the caterpillars, so, the hospital's neonatal unit was soon back to having no functional incubators or devices to support the teeming population of needy neonates. Hence, neonatal mortality rate soared.

The caterpillars would, of course, be informed of the disaster, but they would turn a blind eye to it as the money for it had already been emptied into their private pockets. It could take years before the caterpillars would accommodate another financial appropriation in the budget for this and import enough replacement incubators. And the two- or three-yearly vicious circle of budget-cuts-importation-failure-discard-and re-budget continued. The caterpillars could not appreciate that neonatal incubator intervention was both culture- and climate-sensitive. They completely swallowed the application techniques of the producing countries without paying attention to Nigerian peculiarities. They failed to understand that the foreign manufacturers were primarily interested in Nigeria for business, so they would never advise the brainless Nigerian caterpillars to look inwards and think.

It would be foolish of the foreigner to shoot himself in the foot. The colonising white man made the foolish caterpillars believe that the African brain was not mature enough to create incubator technology that could save the African neonates, so the babies continued to die. The indices of mortality were never improving, irrespective of the money being spent. What response could the Western man give to Nigeria? This was simple: 'If you do not have enough money to purchase more incubators, then try kangaroo mother care'.

Truthfully, the foreign partners showed some level of compassion in daring to return some of their booty from Africa in the name of 'foreign aid'. They were however happier that more and more 'brainwashed' Africans remained the ruling class in the 'dark' continent. The imperialist western countries such as the USA and Great Britain would ensure that Nigeria and, in fact, Africa remained technological beggars, so it was imperative that the Western countries should not allow intelligent Nigerians to become politically powerful. This would not work in favour of their game of stealing million dollars with the left hand during the night, but giving a cent of foreign aid with the right hand during the day.

How dare they suggest that Africans should use KMC instead of proper incubator technology? In fact, the caterpillars provided the opportunity for foreign experts to come and teach the Nigerian mothers how to put their babies on their chests to warm them up through their skin contact – and they called this 'international collaboration achievement'. Brilliant, isn't it? Okay, KMC was very good, in fact, excellent in all cases for the care of the newborn – BUT ONLY IN AFRICA! If KMC could effectively replace proper incubator care for all classes of premature neonates, then it would be fully applied in the teaching hospitals of the USA and Britain. However, these top global centres knew better than to warm a 1000g neonate via the KMC technique. It was a wise concept to the Nigerian caterpillars and African brain-washed leaders because the light-skinned foreign man told them so.

There was however more to this than met the eye. The caterpillars could have welcomed the foreign man's so-called gift aid, but not relented in devising home-grown technologies to reduce their overdependence on imported technologies. They could have supported and encouraged independent researchers whose products might be able to compete with these expensive and hard-to-maintain foreign devices. Homegrown neonatal devices could have been sustainable, readily available and easily maintainable by the local people. These would have in no small measure helped to sustain the availability of proper and scientific incubator application to save the large numbers of neonates that died from thermal distress, both hypothermia and hyperthermia.

I often wondered how a country with hundreds of professors of engineering and medicine in multitudes of universities could not apply basic science to develop life-support applications for neonatal practice. The shameless academics appeared on television to blame their failure on lack of practice devices and inability of the government to provide funds for importation of the much-needed medical systems. They waited for the government forever whilst graduating countless numbers of young students who could have been strategically tasked to engage their energetic brains in looking for solutions. They continued to wait until they had squandered the entire quarter of a century set aside to synthesise solutions for the survival of the neonates. What a tragedy! One would ask these arrogant brain-retarded professors: 'What did you do with your so-called research grants at your institutions? Must the government give you money to import another professor's own devices from another country? Wasn't it shameful that you watched neonates die without translating your theories into devices that could have saved them?

Of what use were the universities, teaching hospitals and their professors to the babies who died? It was okay for the professors to complain against the dumb-brained government officials; however, they could have put on their thinking caps to develop homegrown ideas that could help. The teaching institutions could not invent appropriate devices for Nigeria's paediatric and neonatal medicine; hence the neonates died. The professors were unable to self-motivate themselves in translatable research that could have enabled them to question the bad choices of the government – bad policies that led Nigeria to MDG4 failure. They allowed their institutions to be used to generate false scientific data that covered up faulty and fictitious expenditure, and the neonates died. They could not do effective research with any little grant obtained. What kind of research and academic journal papers did the universities produce? Why couldn't their research produce any solutions that could have averted the MDG4 failure? How many of the professors used rigorously generated data to provide evidence for challenging the ineffective ideas wholesomely imported from foreign cultures and climates? Whilst they were busy competing in the pinching exercise with immoral government official, the Nigerian neonates died, and continued to die under their watch.

Entrepreneurship and industry

Nigerian industrialists and entrepreneurs acted in an unconcerned manner. Were they interested? If so, they could have funded willing researchers at the universities to develop possible ideas that were indigenous and effective. Good ideas and products could always compete in a seemingly unregulated market such as Nigeria's medical technology market. Lazy competitors would always complain of an unequal playing field. They would want to do nothing unless the government stopped or suspended foreign competition. This was a dangerous mindset, as the presence of these foreign products could be a positive stimulant to challenge the effectiveness of local products. The first action for local industry should have been to innovate or collaborate with academia to innovate attractive alternatives – products that would be equally effective or better than the imported 'money-guzzling' brands. They should have accomplished this before asking the government to justify their craving for the importation of medical devices. So the entrepreneurs and industrialists failed the Nigerian neonates and also contributed to sending many to their untimely graves. This also includes the marketers of hospital and clinical equipment, many of whom were financially capable of funding and motivating budding designers and researchers. They failed to so invest meaningfully in Nigeria's technological development, but rather preferred to flood the market with imported goods, many of compromised quality. The Nigerian marketers, the entrepreneurs and the industrialists, all looked the other way whilst the Nigerian neonates died.

A system of periodic review of all the 'true' data being collected from across the country could have genuinely helped Nigeria as a nation to adjust, rethink her strategies and stay on course for the MDG4 target. Nigeria's caterpillars in the Civil Service and Ministries of Health, however, ignored clear indications of impending failure.

Mortalities of the various components of under-five years child health were widely published in terms of neonates, infants and older U5s. This was enough to remind the caterpillars that Nigerian neonates were not surviving in appropriate proportion as MDG4 raced towards 2015. Huge numbers of neonatal deaths at Nigeria's various tertiary centres were enough to trigger the alarm of failure in the hard-of-hearing caterpillars. The alarms went off through scientific and journal paper publications; I sounded these alarms, some other people also did. However, these fell on deaf ears for those in control of government resources. The clear warnings being sounded by me and the few others, who refused to be part of the crippling corruption, were proudly ignored by the caterpillars. They were instead busy spreading the lies of their fictitious scientific data – promising Nigerians that the country was on course to a successful MDG4.

Year 2015 has come and gone; MDG4 has ended and results published. One might rightly ask: where are the caterpillars that deceived Nigerians and crashed the country's MDG4 dreams? These 'neonatophobic' fellows should now cover their faces in shame and walk away with their amassed financial fortunes stolen from public funds that could have saved millions of babies. To think that these shameless fellows gave up their jobs in honour is to wish the impossible – not in the Nigeria I know!

I can vividly recollect an exclusive invitation to deliver a talk at the Nigerian High Commission in London in the year before end of MDG4. The High Commissioner, all his ministers and diplomatic mission agents were in attendance. In my paper entitled 'My passion, their agony, our loss – premature babies in rural Nigeria deserved to survive,' I warned Nigeria: 'My wealth of practical knowledge of the actual situations at our SCBUs across the entire landscape of the country showed that Nigeria would never meet the MDG4 target.'

Amidst many questions and reactions after my thought-provoking lecture was an audacious comment from an agent. I was challenged to my face at that meeting by this Federal Government Medical Attaché to the High Commission, who insisted that Nigeria was on course to success based on the data he was getting from Abuja. He spoke vehemently based on what the caterpillars at Abuja were telling him, whereas I spoke based on clear evidence of true data collected through my many research groups across the country.

I had a good sense of humour and could often throw in surprises. I had been quietly working for many years, collecting my data as I predicted the caterpillars early enough. The end of the 25-years MDG4 was less than two years away, and I was very sure Nigerians had been fooled. The challenge from the Medical Attaché needed a forceful response.

In my reaction to the comment, I said: 'The challenge was baseless given the credentials of my neonatal research and its national coverage, as was evident from my talk'.

I wanted the audience to feel the gravity of my conviction of the impending MDG4 failure, so I openly pledged to destroy my PhD certificate from the prestigious Royal University if Nigeria met the MDG4 target by the end of 2015. I was not presumptuous; in tears, I begged Nigerians to reject the selfishness and love of money that were clear trade-off factors against the innocent lives of the neonates. The year 2015 (end of MDG4) had come and gone, and they now knew better who the liar really was.

Vulnerability and death rate amongst the under-fives decreased with age; hence, more resources and research should have been channelled towards the younger categories – the neonates. What did the Nigerian caterpillars do with WHO information such as: '40% of U5 mortality was being contributed by the neonates'? Why did they not realise that unabated high neonatal mortality would spell doom for the entire MDG4 project? I guess the academics and professors never really realised this in their active minds; to them, this was just bookish knowledge. What did they do to avoid the disaster? If they did anything at all, why were their actions so weak that neonatal mortality rate remained high till the very end, and hence forced MDG4 into a colossal failure?

My strategies

From the very outset, my dream was to decisively tackle the problem of high neonatal mortality as a project with national coverage, whether as one man or otherwise. What I did not realise initially was the importance of my ambitious project. I had no idea of the threats posed by Nigerian adults themselves, whose neonates were being neglected to die needlessly. Nigeria was such a large country with a population of over 185 million people, across six distinct regions divided by language, culture, religion and social values. The land area spanned a whopping 911,000 square kilometres, with poor road networks, deadly airport facilities and dangerously paved roads linking the various cities. These factors were a very powerful impediment to easy societal transformation in Nigeria, yet governments never dared to sincerely tackle them. Functionaries of succeeding governments rather used these factors as guise for mismanaging funds through unlimited looting of the national treasury. They made budgetary allocations year by year and squandered the money each year without solving the problems. These ugly factors were all there like smouldering logs of wood, producing fumes that suffocated the very nationhood of Africa's most populous country.

I was a true Nigerian, detribalised and extremely skilled in my chosen career. I was prepared to go anywhere in Nigeria, provided an 'open door' of invitation was extended to me, from the far-south city of Calabar to Sokoto and Maiduguri in the far north. I carefully studied people, the SCBU environments and the literature so as to build my own perspective of the neonatal drawbacks, and mapped out my own strategy of tackling the problem, initially as one man. I knew that the problem was a national one, so I never discriminated by denying any section of the country from my outreach. I built a practice that covered the entire country, affecting virtually every state in Nigeria (see Appendix 3, map of spread across Nigeria). How could such a small group of individuals in my setup be able to run an organisation that would be able to make an impact in every part of Nigeria?

I had a lot of thinking to do in order to realise my dream. My strategy to approach the problem through provision of sustainable functional technology and enhancement of SCBU knowledge through teaching could conventionally require a lot of money to fund. I had no external funding agency, no industrial backup or any research grants like other academic researchers at the universities. However, I had to build a practice that would always be available and sustainable to the SCBUs irrespective of where these were located in Nigeria. My new ideas for tackling the problem were considered 'unconventional' as they worked contrary to government's incessant importation of technologies – a strategy that was passionately hated by many Nigerian civil servants at the procurement departments otherwise here referred to as the caterpillars. Imports and endless purchases of technology from every part of the world offered civil servants easy routes for looting government money that were meant for solving the neonatal problems.

I insisted that Nigeria must find a way of locally developing some of the solutions that could work, addressing the country's global technology need. The corrupt Ministry of Health functionaries would not support my course of action for this obvious reason. After the launch of my first set of made-in-Nigeria neonatal devices in 1999, the President of the Nigerian Society of Engineers (NSE) had enthusiastically promised to relay the good news to the government and the Nigerian President, so as to organise a formal national presentation of the devices. The promise disappeared into thin air as no one paid any attention to the NSE because it did not provide a good avenue for selfish gains, perhaps. I was abandoned by the NSE and the National Postgraduate Medical College of Nigeria (NPMCN), whose officials for Paediatrics Division also paid a visit to inspect the newly devised neonatal systems at about the same time as the NSE. The NSE and NPMCN could not win government attention and, hence, completely abandoned me and my wild dream of doing the impossible. They treated my ideas with contempt and declared them a 'daydream', inconsequential and of no value. I was little known and had no others to speak for me; however, I was sure the bullying government functionaries were wrong in their approach. How I wished there could be an open contest to challenge who was right.

The entire landscape of national health coverage was the battlefield. How could I find a way of initiating my own battles upon it, smuggle my techniques across the country, quietly measure and publish my outcomes and comparatively assess them against the parallel national techniques? If this could happen in favour of my ideas, I would silence the caterpillars forever, shame them and win victory for the Nigerian neonates.

I was sorely disappointed by the abandonment of NSE and the Paediatrics Division of NPMCN. However, I refused to give up. In order to actualise my dreams, I would have to go 'underground' and work harder to challenge the intelligence of these national caterpillars. I would depend on the desperate Chief Medical Directors – the very few of them who genuinely wanted to lower neonatal mortality at their respective hospital centres. I would have to find a way of making my outreach attractive to any willing CMD. My technologies and teaching courses must be affordable, effective and offer clear evidence of lowering neonatal mortality rate. Poor neonatal outcomes orchestrated by many factors, including non-availability of sustainable incubator intervention, was the dreaded problem of every CMD. It would be a huge achievement if any CMD could demonstrate an appreciable increase in his SCBU's fleet of functional incubators, and sustainably maintain the capacity for his entire tenure in office. It was arguably a near impossibility for any CMD at the time. If I could offer this promise alongside an affordable way of achieving this, surely many of the CMDs would jump at the offer.

My technique must be such that the CMDs would easily assess whether the unconventional applications were effective based on the daily and weekly reports or complaints received from the SCBU. I must devise a technique that could ensure minimum operational costs and overheads, without necessarily compromising on the quality of service. A traditional approach to this kind of setting could be to (1) set up a company, (2) build factories or workshops, (3) hire warehouses, (4) employ technical, clinical, clerical and sales staff, etc. These would all come with huge investments of money which I had no hope of having. Other methods must be devised.

I did not choose the more conventional method of establishing a workshop/factory base, perhaps at one or two locations around the country, and then persuading the hospital executives to move their malfunctioning incubators to the centre for repairs. The mere thought of the costs of transportation of the systems, coupled with the uncertainty of these being successfully fixed, would weaken the resolve of any CMD to give approval for a move.

I decided to opt for an unconventional method involving taking the technology and teaching courses to the premises of each hospital that showed interest. I had never come across or read of this sort of technique previously, but I could not come up with any other model of implementation for my delicate 'underground' moves. How could I implement this kind of idea? It would mean operating a mobile company, with technical workshops that could move from hospital to hospital on service trips. I always believed that achievement of great successes capable of evidence-based demonstrations would depend on quality 'thinking time' to synthesise these solutions. I devised my recycling incubator technology (RIT) and began to move around the inviting tertiary hospitals, reusing the casings and some accessories of the malfunctioning systems and reactivating them with my new operating components. Hospitals were happy to pay the modest costs I charged, as these were often less than 20% of the costs for acquiring or importing brand new replacements. Moreover, the new technique was making it possible to use old and abandoned equipment to restore the hospital's functional incubators. The outcomes were not limited to the increased intervention capacity or reduced mortality; the technique helped to evacuate the abandoned carcasses that littered the hospital, breeding rodents and mosquitoes, hence minimising environmental polution. It was a 'win win' strategy.

The hospitals loved these outcomes and hence were happy to pay the charges. I had no funding or promise of funding from any global health agency, or any grant awards, despite my numerous success stories. I would, however, not compromise on research investigations for advancing the understanding of possible frugal techniques and procedures. I must prudently manage consultancy payments I received from the hospitals so as to save the money needed for funding these research projects. I also worked out how I might apply payments of services from the benefiting teaching hospitals to further expand the reach of my services across Nigeria, and also drive a teaching method that could improve the understanding of doctors and nurses who worked at the neonatal care centres.

I spent more time in thinking how to perfect my money-saving techniques. I believed that the small amount of income from the teaching hospitals could go a long way if I could invest in quality thinking time; I often said it was 80% thinking time and 20% funding-raising time.

A transportation strategy

My friendship with the CMDs' club gave me a transportation strategy. I used the club to build a unification bond across member hospitals, such that one hospital paid indirect transport assistance to reach the next hospital, as will be explained later. The Nigerian federal tertiary hospitals were distributed across the country so that every state had at least one tertiary hospital and in few cases another state-owned one which handled neonatal referral cases.

When I got an invitation from any needy hospital, I first carried out an assessment/advice visit, for a first-hand inspection and understanding of the true state of the incubator systems at the centre in order to generate a reliable system restoration plan. I would then produce a cost estimate for the hospital management to work with. This exercise could take as much as three days to complete, due to the great distances between the Nigerian state capitals where these federal hospitals were often located. This notwithstanding, I preferred to carry out this assessment free of charge in order to motivate the hospitals. This gesture of up to three days' free service might have helped to endear me to some CMDs, who saw it as a sign of technical strength and confidence. I made this journey with an organised toolbox referred to as 'the Emergency Box', containing various tools I would require to make system diagnoses to ascertain faults.

The second trip would normally be for the execution of the project if my quotation was accepted by the hospital management. The CMDs and the Works Departments loved my style of carrying out the job on hospital premises as opposed to the popular repair convention where contractors removed the systems to their local workshops, out of sight of hospital staff. Hospitals had lost many valuable items of equipment as some of the technicians mixed them up with items from elsewhere. Some machines were unaccounted for afterwards because they stayed too long in the local workshops on the pretence of 'looking for spare parts'. This was a frustrating scenario that ruled the era of medical equipment maintenance at the Nigerian hospitals before I stepped in.

One CMD once said to me: 'We have ten incubators, and all of them are malfunctioning, some for many years. You have come from far eastern Nigeria to the north, so how are you going to travel with this massive load of equipment to your workshop in the east and how are we sure our systems won't get lost?' It was such a relief for many that the incubators did not need to be taken away any more. 'This is a brilliant idea and technique, who would fault this?' responded the excited CMD.

The conventional idea of a 'mobile workshop' could easily be pictured as a van with the interior converted into shelves, holding workshop tools and machinery. Sustainability of such a workshop would be difficult to achieve in Nigeria, considering the need for a large vehicle that could cover long distances with the employment of a permanent driver. Moreover, breakdown risks on impassable Nigerian roads were capable of frustrating the system. In order to ensure minimum overheads, I completely avoided ownership of a motor vehicle to operate my mobile workshop. I opted for the idea of using notable transport companies in Nigeria such as ABC Transport Ltd and Peace Mass Transit Ltd in moving a total of 10 Stanley Pro-mobile tool chests around the country. All necessary spare parts and mobile work tools were arranged in the chests, appropriately numbered 1-9, plus an 'emergency box'. Over 5000 pieces of tools and items of incubator spare parts were stored and moved in these boxes.

I appointed a Field Manager amongst my permanent technical staff and he remained in charge of the movement of these boxes at all times. Hospitals allocated temporary spaces for the storage of the boxes, and provided a section of work area as I carried out my technical routines on the incubators during each consultancy visit. In order to maintain a standard of operation, every hospital signed an agreement with my consultancy organisation – Newlife Campaigns for Africa (NCA). The agreement ensured that the hospital was responsible for the movement of the work boxes between the hospital and the appropriate Motor Park or airport at arrival and departure. When preferable, the agreement also mandated each hospital to move the boxes and the team of my support staff to the next hospital in the schedule. This coordinated pattern of movement of materials and human support continued until the last hospital in the schedule of each quarter-yearly tour had been visited. At the end of each consulting tour or during off-duty periods, the boxes were moved into a donated storage space at Lagos. Non-routinely utilised items of extra spare parts or modules for construction and substitution of machine parts were left at the Lagos storage until when needed. These were easily sent wherever needed – even when the field team were already at work – through the coordinated operations of a Logistics Manager stationed at Lagos and an independent cargo operator at Lagos Airport. Spare parts were easily despatched to the nearest local airports for collection by the hospital's vehicle/driver attached to me during each consulting period. The mobile workshop was thus managed with minimal hitches, operating very efficiently, as many of the CMDs gave me their maximum cooperation to operate this technique.

The 'Nigerian character,' as many would say, also reared its head to frustrate the idea. Quite a few CMDs, who thought that it was okay to cheat others in order to survive, played tricks on the operation of this method. Notorious among them were the CMDs of Owerri Federal Infirmary and Gwagwalada Medical Centre. Each of them would always complain of not having enough vehicles for their day-to-day operation, pleading to be excused from that clause of the agreement during most of the routine tours. I continued with the method, since there were only two or three such ungrateful CMDs at each time. I found alternative ways to hire private transport at such times in order not to disrupt the tour. The most annoying aspect of this was that these supposedly happy CMDs signed the consultancy agreements, accepting the discounts that pertained to materials' transport. They would clearly say that they remembered that aspect of the agreement, yet insisted on cheating. This brewed frustrations that often made me feel like withdrawing my consultancy from such hospitals.

On a few occasions, this was one of the many reasons that led to my refusal to renew expired agreements. Worst amongst the culprits were the CMDs who subtly expected some kind of gratification but failed to achieve this owing to my unyielding stance. As a matter of principle, I was not prepared to initiate legal action against any defaulting hospital or CMD as I viewed that as a distraction from my work to save the neonates. I would let the 'stubborn' CMDs cheat me by not fighting back when they withheld my pay or neglected any aspect of the legal Agreement. My revenge was to quietly withdraw my consultancy, thereby bringing back the ugly days of embarrassingly high neonatal mortality to such hospitals. This kind of disrespect for the contents of agreement documents was barbaric.

I tried to epitomise national patriotism by combing through every part of Nigeria, dismissing the fears of unsafe roads, poorly-maintained vehicles, the rampaging of hoodlums and terrorist activities of kidnappers and, of Boko Haram Islamic terrorists in the north. However, I remained conscious of the risks I was taking in all my journeys. I realised that being equally a British national would not prevent the dangers I was exposed to, but might rather exacerbate them. My African street wisdom kicked in almost unconsciously every time I approached International Arrivals at Murtala Mohammed Airport, Lagos, my usual port of entry. I understood I could be duped on the street or robbed at the hotels or fall victim to food poisoning if I unknowingly got into the wrong hands or the wrong places. The three aspects – food, transport and accommodation safety – were not to be compromised, as these could easily distract my team from the main technical and clinical work at the SCBU being visited.

The health and safety of all team members were equally important to me, just like that of the neonates we had come to save. I often opined that the best custodians to guarantee the most appropriate and safe accommodation, feeding and local transport were the hospital management itself, as hospital staff were expected to know their various local environments better than any visitor. Hence, the hospital legal agreement documents provided consultancy discounts in place of mandatory responsibilities for these three needs.

Support staff

I knew that personnel management and staff benefit costs could easily cause my overheads to spiral out of control. I needed enough trained staff to cover the effective technical and clinical support I had planned for all the SCBUs under my consultancy. How could this be achieved without adequate funding to cover staff salaries and benefits all year round? The choice of an itinerant workshop services style meant that support staff could only be engaged during the few months when they were out on their routine maintenance tour of the SCBU systems. I perfected a routine of carrying out the services during particular month of each quarter. This essentially meant that all my team members were on field duty for four months only during a service year, leaving them with a whopping eight months of the year when no income was expected. I was hence left with the option of a kind of 'part time' staff employment which could guarantee the availability of the trained personnel during every 'service tour' month. I prioritised the need for staff members to have a second gainful job that could keep them engaged for the eight months when they were off duty – preferably a self-employed business venture where such staff would have full control of their scheduling.

I operated with three cadres of supporting staff and professionals; namely the Central Technical Staff (CTS) that travelled through all SCBU cities with me during routine service-tour, the Occasional City Assistants who were resident technicians at each city where an SCBU was located and, finally my Collaboration Clinical team of doctors and nurses located at the various SCBUs. I skilfully managed all groups of staff such that everyone was proud to be associated with the great achievements of 'Newlife Campaigns for Africa'.

The mobile workshop was pitched at each benefiting hospital twice a year – six months in between each routine visit. Therefore all the hospitals benefiting from the consultancy were divided into two groups in equal numbers: group A visited during a month of the first quarter and 3rd quarter and, group B during 2nd quarter and the 4th quarter. The members of the central technical staff team were carefully recruited, ensuring that they did not significantly dislike travelling far by road or air.

Every CTS was allowed to operate an independent service tour account, referred to as the 'imprest' account. I periodically transferred cash into each staff member's bank account to fund it. This designated account independently empowered every employee and ensured readily available cash to spend accountably to prevent factors that might limit prompt completion of any task during the tour. Every staff member has to come to terms with my golden rule for the actualisation of service-tour mandates – 'no excuses for failures'. I asked every staff member to learn to read the signs that could warn of the failure of assignment targets and to send adequately-timed warnings to the appropriate line manager or to me if such factors were out of the immediate control of the employee. Both occasional and CT staff were well-educated on their limits of decision making to avoid unauthorised steps that could endanger the lives of the neonates or the SCBU local staff.

I ensured that all reasonable expenditure incurred by my staff was paid through the imprest account. All were required to submit expenses at the end of each service tour. A standard Microsoft Excel spreadsheet template document referred to as 'the cash-manager' was developed for book keeping. My staff found this tool very useful, one of them commenting: 'The cash-manager is quite magical. It removes the nightmare of doing acceptable accounting for all my expenses; I love it'.

I designed research projects that could fit into applicable research skills for resident doctors working with me. I motivated them to completion of such projects, ensuring good quality data for international journal publications. I tried to identify clinical and nursing staff members of the SCBUs who could be inspired, and encouraged them to collaborate in the research, especially the aspect of generating or extracting the clinical outcome data using the various study proformas I designed for each research operation. This method also enhanced the teaching aspect of my work as I trained the practitioners on the various 'unconventional' approaches I was devising. There was no direct cash remuneration for the clinicians and nurses; they were paid agreed professional charges whenever I co-opted anyone as a resource person in a training course for a different SCBU other than his or her own centre. All participating medics benefited through co-authorships of the resulting conference and journal articles we published. Co-authorship of investigations with me was taken with pride among the doctors and nurses because of the high quality rating associated with my works. Our study-anchoring clinicians and nurses were excellent Nigerians that served the neonates willingly and sacrificially.

Thus, the overall minimally affordable charges that I made the hospitals pay for the services I rendered was prudently managed in order to maintain a decent size of workforce that were happy to respond to action as soon as they were notified. My team never defaulted in showing up for scheduled routine services at any SCBU throughout the country. I completely rejected to give excuses such as 'there were no ready staff to be despatched for the routine services'. In fact, I was physically present to lead the team during all routine service tours. I did everything within my ability, ensuring that every staff member was happy.

CHAPTER 12

THE COMPONENT MANUFACTURER FROM THE LAGOS BACK STREETS

✦✦✦✦✦✦✦

The primary assignment the hospitals desired of the Newlife Campaigns team was the creation of recycled incubator (RIT) systems out of any malfunctioning incubators at the participating SCBU centre. Subsequent to this was the routine maintenance of all the functional incubators and the other thermoneutral systems at the Unit, hence preventing system break-down due to avoidable causes. I understood that a sustainable system maintenance culture would be hard to achieve without availability of spare parts. I personally designed or reconfigured the numerous RIT system components by myself. These were crafted so as to make them reproducible within the limited capabilities of ordinary 'street' artisans.

Spare parts production

Nigerian artisans are skilful self-employed entrepreneurs who owned small workshops and produced goods and services that were consumed locally. Over the years of my consultancy services, I remained on the lookout for talented artisans. I inspected the machinery and tools available at the artisan's workshop and the quality of his finished products. Once satisfied with these, I negotiated with the artisan, educating him on the techniques to adopt in the production of the particular 'incubator part' of interest. I used practical demonstrations and guided them to produce samples. Successful artisans were awarded contracts for the production of given quantities of the spare part whenever my team ran out of supplies. I had artisans in Lagos and Port Harcourt who produced various Perspex components that served in different models of my RIT systems. The artisan for fabric components was stationed in Owerri and Jos. I had co-opted welders and painters in the cities where the SCBUs were located. All these artisans owned and operated their workshops, but they gave priority to Newlife Campaigns' components as soon as requisitions were sent in.

Shola boy

Lagos is perhaps the most densely-populated part of Nigeria. Formerly the capital, it was the home of the busiest international airport and seaport in the country. A large number of signs displaying public and private enterprises hung indiscriminately on the walls of buildings and balconies, and many others were erected on poles beside the gutters that lined the streets. The streets of Lagos had no clear pedestrian walkways; one had to make conscious efforts to avoid cars whizzing past at unreasonable speeds. There was loud music coming from virtually every shop along the streets, which added to the noise coming from mini power generators beside every shop. The generators continuously pumped large amounts of carbon monoxide into the street, polluting the immediate vicinity. I wondered how people survived in a typically busy commercial street.

One of my old school friends, a Lagos resident, drove me out for a drink around the Ikeja area of Lagos through one of the busy commercial streets. My eyes caught a signpost with the message: 'SHOLABOY – fantastic at plastic signwriting'. I asked my friend to stop and went into the workshop to inquire about the work carried out by this Sholaboy.

'I really want to talk with the main man behind these plastic signs,' I said to the young man inside.

'I am the one, sir,' he replied. His name was Lekan, but he was also Sholaboy.

'Okay, I like your work and would like to introduce you to other products that you can produce for me using this kind of Perspex. I can see that you have great skills with Perspex. I only need to teach you how to make the various items I have designed.'

'That is most welcomed sir. I appreciate it sir,' responded Sholaboy.

In the days and weeks that followed, I spent a lot of time taking Sholaboy through the patterns, precision, finishing and overall quality of five different shapes of Perspex components for incubator spare parts. Sholaboy never knew what these items were used for or where exactly they were being taken to in the first two years of his being co-opted into my Occasional staff team.

Sholaboy was a respectful man who diligently carried out all job requisitions, delivering them promptly. He was quick to understand and responded positively to my high standards of quality and promptness in service delivery. Sholaboy was honest; he readily discussed difficult situations relating to his job with me and so avoided disappointments and the need to give excuses for failures. Sholaboy had minimal education but did not find it very hard to understand technical instructions, carrying these out to the last detail. He played a big role in helping me to actualise the assignment of saving the neonates. I also had great respect for him.

Sholaboy grew in confidence on the job and interactions with me and some of my other team members. One day he asked me: 'Sir, hope you don't mind, but I wish to know what you do with these tiny pieces of plastic that I produce for you as I am becoming very curious?'

'Sure, I don't mind. It is not a secret but what if I don't tell you?' I replied.

'Nothing would happen sir, as I enjoy being part of whatever good job you are doing with these. I only perceive that I may be part of a great solution that is addressing an urgent need in the society without knowing it,' Sholaboy politely responded. I was touched by his soft spoken response, delivered with a voice full of respect and submission. 'Okay then,' I said: 'I will take you to the very place where your products are being used for a great job, but you must be prepared for it, okay?'

'I would appreciate that, sir,' said Sholaboy.

Newlife Campaigns' outreach to Lagos Tertiary Hospital (LTH) yielded fantastic results between 2007 and 2014. The great support received from Akin, the gentleman CMD, enabled Newlife Campaigns for Africa to grow the incubator fleet at the SCBU of the LTH into one of the largest capacity amongst all Nigerian SCBUs. This numbered over thirty functional incubators and resuscitaires during the period. My team would normally spend over ten days at LTH during each routine service visit due to its size and high patient turnover. Large quantities of breakable Perspex components were frequently replaced during the service routine.

I took Sholaboy to the 'gowning' room, at the entrance of the SCBU and handed him a gown, scrub and head cover. I picked up another set for myself and said: 'Watch how I dress up in these materials and do the same'. We stepped into the Unit and were aptly greeted by much high-pitched crying of tiny neonates from all corners of the Unit.

'Sir, do they deliver babies here?' asked Sholaboy in a shaky voice.

'No, don't be frightened. We look after premature and sick newborn babies here to stop them from dying. We put them inside machines called incubators that provide them with adequate humidification and warmth whilst we treat them,' I replied.

We entered the main incubator bay, and on seeing many rows of tiny neonates inside incubators, Sholaboy was quick to identify where some of his Perspex products fitted on the peripheries of the incubators. He looked into a few incubators.

'Sir, I have never seen babies as tiny as these in my life. Do they really survive?'

'Yes, many of them will survive provided there are available functional incubators to do the indispensable job of providing them with an appropriate womblike environment at this stage of their lives,' I replied.

'And my plastic, how does it help?' questioned Sholaboy.

'The incubators won't function properly if those Perspex components you make for me were removed, so they are actually life-saving components,' I replied.

As we walked back to the reception area, Sholaboy remained speechless as though shocked by what he had seen. He removed his gown, looked me in the eye and said: 'Thank you sir for showing me round. I actually was not prepared for what I saw. I now know how important my work is and why I must always continue to prioritise the production of these components whenever you place an order. I wish to thank you again for getting me involved'. Sholaboy remains a very important artisan member of Newlife Campaigns for Africa.

A number of young men joined my neonatal survival crusade at various times. It was often difficult to identify prospective employees who possessed the combinations of intelligence, hard work and enduring strength for the vast amount of travelling required for this work. I understood that it would take a true love for the neonates for any young man to remain long as an active staff member. Many new employees struggled with the whole idea of the work after being employed, so they never lasted beyond a year before resigning. Some stayed longer, expecting to somehow get rich through the job, but soon became frustrated as they began to discover that it was not the kind of work for the 'get rich quick', so they left the company. A few of the departing staff did not leave quietly. Some duped the organisation by disappearing with some of the materials; others were properly relieved of their duties when their unruly behaviour at the SCBUs became an embarrassment to the organisation. I always ensured a peaceful departure. I never bothered to prosecute those that stole from the organisation, as I considered this a distraction. I always had huge faith in the ability of my God to help me bounce back, replacing whatever had been lost.

It was often nightmarish for me whenever a support staff member started to behave in a manner that showed discontent or the possibility of being dropped from the team. This was because of the great effort, time and resources it would normally take to train a replacement. I would work hard to resolve conflicts and succeeded at times, but at other times I failed, and was left with the only option of sacking the employee.

In addition to paying workers promptly, I did not stint on the praise I gave to high-performing staff. I believed that showing due respect and diligent acknowledgement of good performance encouraged workers to excel all the more. This theory was not completely correct, as evidenced by the outcome of some characters such as Mr Ochulo and Mr Amos. Mr Ochulo was a university graduate in Electrical Engineering but could hardly speak or write comprehensible English. It was very easy to mistake him for someone who had not attended secondary school, due to his poor writing and speaking skills. He was a typical example of the poor quality of graduates from some Nigerian universities, especially those from notable parts of the country. Mr Ochulo was however, very hard working; he had no problems travelling the vast distances of the service tour, being in charge of the work boxes. His ability to withstand long hours of work and his promptness at delivering set goals made up for his other shortcomings. He was soon encouraged with promotion for his hard work, but soon after this he began to become unruly, taking the law into his own hands. He began to apply wrong initiatives to deliberately disobey clear instructions and the manner of work at the SCBU. As the field manager, he could not effectively manage the other support staff working under him. He indiscriminately raised his voice in the SCBUs and shouted at his staff, thereby often distracting other clinical and nursing groups working there.

I wondered where all this ugly behaviour was coming from, having worked with Mr Ochulo for nearly four years without noticing them. I asked him to explain his actions a number of times, and was sad that I might end up having to sack Mr Ochulo.

Then came a fateful day when, whilst consulting at the Benin City Federal Hospital, I approached the SCBU to commence my 'ward round' but was disappointed to hear Mr Ochulo's voice from a distance. I was greeted with the sad face of Mr Omenka, one of my CT staff, who was assisting Mr Ochulo.

'Can you, without delay, explain what is going on here, and why you have such a sad face?' I demanded from Mr Omenka.

'Sir, I have been carefully following all the instructions that my manager gave to me but he seemed to get offended with me every inch of the way. I pleaded with him to stop insulting and shouting at me but he refused. Just before you stepped in, he even attempted to hit me, threatening to stab me with a screwdriver.' Mr Omenka was sobbing as he replied.

I was disappointed when Mr Ochulo's defence turned out to be very weak: 'Sir, I only said I go 'chook' you with this thing, only for joke I said it'.

'You did threaten to stab him – right inside the SCBU, right? Do you take this place for a motor park?' I asked in anger. I was thrown into turmoil, since Mr Ochulo was clearly posing a great danger to the SCBUs. It became imperative that arrangements must begin for the replacement of Mr Ochulo before it became too late for the next Newlife Campaigns maintenance tour. Mr Ochulo knew that his position in the organisation was very important, and that none of his junior colleagues could possibly operate in his position at a short notice, so he imagined it was not possible to sack him. He even made a demand for a salary increase. Although this was granted it did little to encourage him to be good. In fact it appeared that the more he was encouraged with respect, the worse he became.

Finally, I consulted all the honorary directors of Newlife Campaigns for Africa, presenting Mr Ochulo's attitudes. The directors voiced their concern and demanded his immediate dismissal.

There were two other high-profile departures of senior staff members whose actions could be interpreted as biting the hand that fed them. Mr Amos, Assistant Field Manager, had two opportunities, but his wicked heart acted against him. His case was similar to Ochulo's, except that he initially left on his own without formal notification to NCA management. He had worked with Newlife Campaigns for nearly five years, rising in rank from the initial post of Field Assistant. Mr Amos was hard working, which endeared him to me, being treated like my own brother. The company assisted him with finance and housing support to alleviate the sudden pressure he encountered after marriage. It was a shock to the NCA management when Mr Amos failed to return to work after all this, walking away with the loans he had received and other property of Newlife Campaigns.

Disdains and doubts

Northeast Nigeria, the year 2011: my vibrant research team at the Ilorin Special Care Baby Unit (SCBU) had concluded a study on the aetiology of a climate-driven neonatal morbidity condition known as 'evening fever syndrome' (EFS). EFS was believed to affect up to 70% of inmates in any SCBU in Nigeria, especially in northern Nigeria where ambient temperatures could reach a staggering 47 degrees Celsius. I would not stop until I had synthesised a functional solution to minimise or eradicate EFS and end the worsening high neonatal morbidity due to the contributions of this condition. I planned to initiate another research study that could test materials, and subsequently develop an effective antidote to evening-fever syndrome in the neonate. The best geographical location for the citing of the study was northeast Nigeria, where the high ambient temperature was perfect for such work. This was the period of bloody warfare and terroristic rampaging of northern Nigeria by the ruthless Boko Haram terror organisation. There were daily occurrences of bombing raids by Boko Haram and many professionals fled this region of Nigeria. It was risky to go to the north – in fact, many people would turn down any assignment that would send them there, especially the northeast state of Yobe, about the hottest war zone at the time. I issued an open invitation to all the Chief Medical Directors of the hospitals under my consultancy, asking for whoever was prepared to collaborate to anchor the research to find a solution for the disabling EFS. All the CMDs declined except one – the nobleman Bellowa of Nguru Federal Tertiary hospital in Yobe State!

Dr Bellowa was doubtful that I would accept his offer for the use of his hospital centre for the study due to the war. He was pleasantly surprised when he received my acceptance letter. The research work was completed and the findings published after three years of concerted work. This attracted invitations to conferences for the dissemination of the scientific information. Among the many organisations where the research took centre stage for discussion was the World Health Organisation Geneva, the 12th World Congress on Medical Devices. I had just finished an electrifying plenary presentation on evening fever syndrome and its antidote as researched and developed by my group in the small town of Nguru in Yobe State Nigeria. I tied my talk in with a global challenge to Africans and other low-income countries, motivating them to 'flex up' their God-given brains to innovate: 'You understand your local environments better than any foreigner. Do not be deceived because you have got brains; put them to work to synthesize the technologies that could work perfectly for your small local environments and economies,' I declared. My story of the intense Nguru work was jaw-dropping. This generated much response at the Plenary Session of the World Congress. Reactions, questions and contributions were pouring in from delegates, and my conclusion was rewarded with a standing ovation.

Unknown to me, among the huge crowd that attended the plenary session was a Nigerian government delegate, Ms Evelyn, a staff member of the Nigerian Drug Administration Commission (NUZDAC), who neither asked a question nor made any reaction to a presentation that sounded bogus to her. She thought this could not have happened in her own country during this period in history. She doubted my claims for obvious reasons. Many other delegates who could not ask their questions due to lack of time during the session lined up in a small group at the end of the session to obtain my reactions to their questions. The line was long, the people were patiently taking their turn, and I was happy to ensure that I listened to every one of them. As this went on, I took notice of this black lady and hoped she would be patient enough for her turn to field-in her questions or reactions.

Finally, it was Ms Evelyn's turn. 'What an electrifying presentation you just gave, it was quite educative,' she said. 'I am from Nigeria and I work for NUZDAC – not sure if you know the organisation from your many travels to Nigeria?'

'Yes, I do,' I replied.

Evelyn continued in a lowered voice: 'I had difficulty accepting the authenticity of the research, especially when you said it was done in Yobe State between 2011 and 2013,' she said. I immediately sensed why this question was coming, so I quickly made a request: 'sorry madam, can you speak a bit louder and repeat your question as these other fellows may benefit from it, please?' I requested. Ms Evelyn repeated her question.

'Thank you for your rightful doubts,' I began as I looked around the other listeners: 'Ladies and gentlemen, I am sure this question, or should I say doubt, has come about because Yobe State was and still is a no-go area for safety reasons due to incessant warfare and the bombings raids of the Boko Haram terrorist organisation. Please madam, correct me if I am wrong.'

'You are absolutely right. This is the reason I wondered how you could claim the execution of this project at the time you indicated. I know that people were even afraid to fly to places like Kano, let alone driving the long hours to Yobe, the most dangerous area. You created the impression that you supervised the work on site yourself. Did you really do this, or were people collecting data and sending it to you in England?'

I could see the interest as everyone around seemed to be curiously awaiting an answer. 'Yes, I did supervise the work in person. The terrors of Boko Haram did not stop me. I was always at my laboratory at Nguru for up to five days in each quarter. Going the extra mile to achieve the impossible is where my strength and joy lie. I love to push the boundaries of adversity to save the neonates. As a human being, I feel the tension during the planning for my trips due to fear of terrorists everywhere in Nigeria, not just the northern part, but the moment I set out on the journey I was not bothered about the dangers any more. I moved carefully but concentrated on the job, powering on all cylinders until I had fulfilled the purpose of the trip. And I tell you, this is what Africans and similar economies need to do to escape from their backwardness and over-reliance on Western technologies,' I concluded, to the admiration of my listeners.

Ms Evelyn of NUZDAC must not be singled out as the only coward in the battle to save Nigerian patients. She was a Nigerian senior civil servant who lived in Lagos in south-western Nigeria with her family but worked at Abuja in north central Nigeria. So she squandered useful funds commuting every week between Lagos and Abuja by air, staying in hotels. She was afraid to take up any assignment in supposed 'dangerous' places and was not prepared to relinquish her office position for another willing officer to occupy. The Nigerian civil service, especially in the medical sector, stank with no one to sanitize it. Many other people wondered aloud in my hearing why on earth a supposed important professor would so often risk his life, flying into Lagos from London, immediately flying to the city of Kano – of all places – during this terror period. The very residents of Nguru in Yobe State were afraid to travel to their capital city, Damaturu. Many would not step out to go to Kano city. Everyone was afraid of the rampaging Boko Haram. Yet, this young man would fly into Kano airport and ask for a driver from Nguru to come and pick him up for the four-hour road journey across the deserts of Yobe to the hospital.

Many staff of the hospital argued about my passion for the neonates and wondered if I was genuinely different from the many doctors they had seen. The Chief Medical Director, Bellowa, loved and cherished my commitment. He would often speak about how Nigeria had been blessed as a nation with the personality of Professor Hippolite. The global exposure that my collaboration had brought to the Nguru hospital earned Dr Bellowa a lot of respect from the Nguru people. I was indeed very popular at the Nguru hospital, especially with the construction of the EFS laboratory, which was initially nicknamed 'Hippolite Underground' by the staff of the Works Department of the hospital. My popularity at Nguru earned me many titles at the hospital as people used various nicknames for me, including one that was interpreted as 'Medical Director's white man'. Nguru locals got to know so much about the 'black-skinned white man' who defied all odds to come to rescue poor tiny neonates in town. They wanted to do everything to impress me. They offered to give me a local young lady to serve as my wife whenever I was visiting. I thanked them for their kindness, but respectfully declined the offer as being unnecessary.

The climax of all the appreciation from the Nguru people was a vehement declaration on one occasion when a highly-placed gentleman came to me and said: 'We all pray for you, doctor. No matter how much risk you take for us or our babies, nothing bad will happen to you. Boko Haram cannot harm you because even the neonates are all praying for you until their discharge from the hospital. You do know that, don't you? You know the Islamic position during prayer – we kneel down with the forehead on the floor – this is also the resting position I often see newborn babies in on the ward, so they are all interceding for you too,' he said. Wow! I could not feel any more blessed than when I heard these powerful comments from this man.

At the end of the study, the EFS laboratory was upgraded to a mini-neonatal ward which the hospital formally named after me in appreciation for my contributions. The centre is still called the Hippolite-Nguru Centre for Neonatal Research.

CHAPTER 13

GOD – THE SUPERNATURAL

✦✦✦✦✦✦✦

It had always been my desire to become a university professor some time in my life. My ambition dated back to immediately after graduation from my first MSc degree in Nigeria. In 1991, I applied to the University of Ontario, Canada, for a possible PhD programme. I was required to concisely deliver my one-page 'statement of purpose' for my chosen course and career. I did not hesitate to state: 'I dream of becoming a great intellectual in medical science and a major contributor to the advancement of medical engineering in the world'.

This was easier said than done. There were obviously many difficult obstacles to overcome before such a professorial desire could be accomplished – academics, research, teaching etc. I felt a step closer when I completed my PhD at the Royal University London many years later. My Department at the University was happy to retain me as a research staff member pending any possible opportunity to elevate me to the teaching staff cadre. Quite a few opportunities came, but I was unsuccessful. I did not want to get myself too busy elsewhere as I felt the Royal was the best place to become a professor. I began to come under enormous pressure due to poor earnings which could not sustain me and my family. My job as a research staff member paid well only when there was a research grant. At other times, it was difficult.

I knew that the only way to secure a future that could guarantee my dreams was to obtain a teaching position at the Royal, if this ever became possible. This failed to come as quickly as I hoped. My senior colleagues at the university could not help me any longer as many of them gave excuses, saying that with government restrictions such employment positions should be given to EU or British citizens only – I did not hold British citizenship until much later in my career. My former supervisor, Dr Harry (later Professor Harry), would give promises of securing me a position but would always end up saying: 'sorry, but I couldn't'. All along I was feeling the great impression that God wanted me elsewhere, and not necessarily in the Royal job I was hoping for. I would quickly brush off thoughts of returning to full-time engagement with my neonatal work in Nigeria. I would raise objections in my thoughts: 'I can still accomplish my neonatal work in Nigeria somehow, but I really want to become a Royal professor. There is no road to this ambition from the 'village' hospitals in Nigeria'.

My friends would notice my worries and advise me to

apply to other UK universities for a possible position, but I had no interest in any other UK university. I knew exactly what my torment was – the Nigerian neonates. They haunted me. When I slept, I dreamt about dying neonates, I dreamt about abandoned babies, I dreamt of weeping mothers mourning their dead newborns, I dreamt about frustrated doctors and nurses on neonatal wards – it was neonates, neonates and more neonates. The more time flew past the more frustrated I became, until I could take it no more. I was gradually falling into a state of depression. I came to my senses and recalled how, as I believed, God had orchestrated and masterminded the situations leading up to my ultimate journey to England many years earlier, and how the dramas of my PhD had unfolded afterwards. I finally concluded that it could have been more difficult for the Lord God to uproot me from Nigeria all the way to completing an MSc, PhD and two Diploma degrees at the very expensive Royal University without any financial assistance from anyone.

After days of thought and dialogue in my heart, I began to tell myself: 'Based on divine events that had happened previously in relation to this UK adventure, it should be easy for God to also orchestrate a proper 'teaching' position for me if He wanted to do so'. My new mindset was that God, in His wisdom, had set up these difficulties in order for me to listen to my inner mind. I began to give up my Royal ambitions. The more I pushed my professorial dreams aside in my mind and thought of new strategies for neonatal survival in Nigeria, the more peace of mind I had. I must now listen to the voice of God once again, so I gave up my ambition and redirected my thoughts to Nigeria – to the neonates across the entire country.

I would unleash the full force of the academic and research skills I had learnt at Royal University to push the boundaries of neonatal survival in Nigeria.

The love for excellent research techniques which I learnt under the great Professor Harry followed me all the way as I made new discoveries for neonatal care in Nigeria. I translated these research techniques from orthopaedics to neonatology. These worked perfectly as I applied them to validate my innovations and converted them into academic resources via peer-reviewed journal publications and conferences. I enjoyed this research dimension, as it made me feel I was still relevant in the research and academic world. I loved to impart the knowledge of my discoveries and the emerging outcomes of my care techniques to my collaborating clinicians, nurses and technicians around the hospital across the entire country. Hence, I developed teaching materials, training course modules and certifications for people attending my courses. My paediatrics incubation technique course modules were popular among the hospitals that wanted to improve their neonatal care outcomes, especially as related to temperature control in the newborn.

Soon I grew to become a seasoned teacher, practical demonstrator, course designer and coordinator. I taught postgraduate clinicians, nurses and technicians all over Nigeria. My course enrolments over the twelve years to the publishing of this book stood at a staggering 1,668 candidates plus numerous unofficial course partcipants. I enjoyed the outcomes of my endeavour and never bothered any longer with my initial ambition to become a Royal professor, often telling myself: 'I am happy doing what God wanted me to do; at least, I am still academically relevant in some ways'.

I never knew God's ultimate plans. By the time they were unfolded and I realised where things were heading, I did not hesitate to bow down to worship God. I later corrected my previous convictions by declaring: 'God does not deny His loved ones any good dreams and ambitions – He rather compels His servants to take the proper direction that is capable of maximizing their talents for better results, and yet arriving at the same dreamt ambitions. God never owes anybody anything, and never robs anyone of ambition. He knows the best way to anyone's ambition, and is always pleased to perfectly drive this if allowed to do so. God did it for me. He can do it for anyone. This sums my experience in giving all things up to follow God's own leading.'

Unknown to me, my freelance and independent research, practice, teaching, course development and publications – the things I enjoyed doing – were mounting up towards a future professorial promotion. When I gave up the struggle to be appointed a teaching academic at Royal University, I gave up the professorial ambition as well. It was not possible for somebody to become a professor without being specifically employed as a full-time teaching staff member in a particular university – at least, this was my impression at the time. So, with this in mind, becoming a university professor was a closed chapter. I concentrated in combing all through the Nigerian dangerous terrains doing what I enjoyed – saving the neonates.

My rare patience enabled me to reject the advice from my friends to walk away from Royal University. Many of my friends decried the discrimination of refusing to appoint me to a full-time teaching position, whilst at the same time referring to me as being excellent at my job. 'What a dishonest way to treat someone. Better walk away,' said one of my close friends.

I was hurt to be denied, but it would cost me nothing to remain at the Royal as an unpaid Research Fellow, since my Department at the Royal University had proposed this honorary position to me. I responded to my friend's advice: 'Offending the Royal will cause me more pain as I still wish to keep the senior friends I made there,' I said. 'Walking away from the Royal and burning my bridges might turn out a dangerous thing to do. Who knows, I might walk into a disaster that would require me to run back to take refuge at Royal University in the future, when there would be no bridge for my escape'.

I kept all my friendships, especially my good relationship with my PhD supervisor, Professor Harry. I technically retained the Royal University as my primary base of employment whilst operating as visiting Consultant/Academic at all the over 25 tertiary and university teaching hospitals I worked for in Nigeria at different times. I hated being referred to as a 'contractor' by these institutions. I argued that the meaning of 'contractor' as used at the institutions was far from the duties I performed. Therefore, I required every institution to officially engage me as a 'visiting consultant,' insisting that the clinical, teaching and local research I often led without pay could not be better described. The institutions willingly obliged me. I had so many invitations to national, regional, continental and world conferences to showcase my numerous discoveries and innovations in the field of neonatology. All my abstracts carried the mark of Royal University London as my primary institutional identity. All my journal publications from the researches also carried the Royal as the primary institutional identity. I owed no institution the obligation of publishing in their names; however, I enjoyed publishing in the name of Royal as a give-back to a great and prestigious university that allowed me many open doors. My former PhD supervisor, Professor Harry, had had an incredible career at Royal University ever since he supervised my work. He was a very intelligent and hardworking man, and had an extraordinary passion for his teaching and research. Harry was rewarded with rapid academic promotions. He became a professor at quite a young age, leading many research groups, study centres and laboratories. He went on to become the Head of Bioengineering at the university. Professor Harry was very proud of my achievements as he had followed my progress and the exploits from my Nigerian work. He wanted to make my work more relevant to bioengineering at Royal University.

Professor Harry became the Head of Department at the time when this mattered most to me, especially regarding the credibility of my many works. Professor Harry was an 'angel of the Lord' sent at the right time for the right purpose – he allowed God to use him in extraordinary ways he might not have known. Upon assumption of office of the Head of Bioengineering, Professor Harry did not hesitate to announce the establishment of a 'virtual' Centre for frugal medical technology, appointing me as the volunteer centre operator. This became the local Unit of Bioengineering that anchored my various titles at the Department, making my work more visible.

An Anglo-Nigerian partnership

Harry closely monitored my research activities, my publications and rising global recognitions. He invited me regularly to his office for update reports and operational discussions. I remained loyal and humble before Harry, who remembered the many struggles I had passed through at the Royal: my difficulties as a student under his supervision, my hard work, my research outputs, my frustrations as a self-funded student and an underpaid Research Fellow for many years. Professor Harry resolved to translate whatever outputs or achievements I was gaining, making these as profitable as he could.

I had become a big name across neonatal institutions all over Nigeria and a major scientific contributor on the world stage. It became necessary to articulate a way of harnessing all the resources that had been developed by my Nigeria research. Proposals were suggested to appoint one Nigerian university to a partnership that could allow an organised postgraduate degree for young Nigerians to study my style of medical know-how to leverage capacity-building in the Nigeria healthcare technology.

Professor Harry did not hesitate to take this forward, and quickly called for applications from interested Nigerian universities. Many applied. As a primary condition for collaboration, Professor Harry demanded that the winning Nigerian University must be willing to accept my local involvement at their Nigerian campus: 'Dr Hippolite must be appointed as the academic chair of the collaboration at the Nigeria University,' he demanded. This led to my initial appointment as Professor of Medical Technology by a Nigerian university. I would remain indebted to Professor Harry for being the willing instrument God used in reviving and actualising my forgotten ambition of becoming a university professor. Indeed God does not kill godly ambitions.

'What an excellent win-win solution! Divine solutions can be incredible!' I exclaimed. 'It would have been impossible for me to maintain a Nigeria nationwide consultancy, saving Nigerian neonates, if I initially got a teaching appointment at Royal University London. The student calendar at the Royal would have made it absolutely impossible to make the frequent Nigeria trips that characterised my neonatal consultancy,' I said joyfully upon receiving my letter of appointment as a professor.

God needed me for the neonates, but he did not want to deny me my lifelong ambition to become a university professor. I never saw God's plans from afar; I simply gave mine up for the neonatal survival of African newborns, as God's will and calling, not to become some kind of professor at some top university. God had all along known how He could use me for the neonates through the many rough experiences I would face, but at the end He brought me back to the prime academic title of 'professor' at the peak of my field career. I felt I was dreaming, yet this was real. My position and title of 'Honorary Research Fellow' was retained at the Royal and ran concurrently with my professorial position in Nigeria for another three years.

My continued rising profile on the world stage was quite compelling. Professor Harry's respect at Royal University had also risen tremendously. In two terms of his headship of the Bioengineering Department, he literally transformed the department into the second largest bioengineering department in the world, being second only to United States' Georgia Tech. Harry was yet to raise another topic that would blow me away.

The phone rang. It was Harry: 'Hi Hippolite, I can see you had requested for my secretary to schedule you for a meeting with me. I am incredibly busy at the moment but will surely be free in two weeks from now. Would this timing be okay for you?'

I replied, 'I really understand how busy you can get, Harry. The next two weeks will be tight for me, but I can always adjust to be available for you. It is actually about my Nigerian updates and a few challenges I am having at the moment. These are the things I have in mind to discuss in the meeting.'

Harry told me he had another proposal to discuss with me, but I had no idea of the surprise awaiting me. The private meeting between Harry and me went very well and we discussed my challenges in Nigeria and my new moves to counter some of these. Finally, it was time for Harry to open up the last item on his agenda. 'Right, Hippolite, I have been going through your profile of late,' he said. 'I think I can compile this in a write-up for submission to the Faculty, making a case for your promotion to the rank of professor here,' he said.

'Wow, I didn't see this coming, Harry,' I replied. 'Thank you so much for the thought, but can it be possible, as I have never held a teaching position here?'

'You have delivered thousands of teaching hours in Nigeria for many years now, developed course modules and supervised academic projects as shown by available records, haven't you?' asked Harry. 'Then develop your short CV for me and I will clock in your Nigerian teaching hours and academic developments in my report – just leave the rest to me.'

I was blown away. 'How could we actualise this new position if approved, as I am still busy with my Nigerian job?' I asked.

'The fact is that we are happy at the Department for all you do in the name of the Royal University. There are no plans of withdrawing you from what you are doing so well. Your new professorial title would have a prefix of 'visiting' appended to it to indicate the nature of your new position.'

I was not sure how this could be possible, but I would not joke about it as I trusted Harry's instincts and capabilities. I did not delay in drafting the short CV as requested by Professor Harry. The whole promotion process took six months for Harry's submissions and defence at the Faculty. Then I received a letter in the post from the Human Resources Department, officially appointing me to the senior academic position and title of 'Visiting Professor'. Unbelievable but true!

I was happy with this new development as it spoke volumes for how highly the Royal regarded my personality, my integrity and my research. Unknown to me, records had been broken by this appointment. I became the first Royal academic of Nigerian descent to be appointed a professor. This adds to my earlier records as the first Nigerian PhD in bioengineering and the first Nigerian professor of engineering in medicine. I was grateful to God and to Professor Harry for encouraging me to follow the best and most profitable route to my lifelong ambition to become a professor at a top university.

Many years later as a professor, I made a leisurely visit to one of England's most compelling historic places, one of my few day-trip escapes from my normal busy life for de-stressing and reflection. Several weeks prior to this visit I had encountered some desperate and confused young graduates within my practice. Each of the individual graduates approached me privately for advice on how they might handle the various alternatives for the future of their careers. Each time I would remember my early days at Royal University, and I used my personal experience to do my best in motivating the youngsters. However I found it extremely difficult to communicate how I had left my future in God's hands to navigate me through life.

My stories often sounded unreal to the graduate students. They understood that I had been an academic success who could inspire them, but there was something not quite 'conventional' about my career. Johnny loved to listen to my advice, but still feared things might turn out badly in his own case. It was unhelpful to toy with the smartness of these youngsters. Johnny once asked: 'Was it not a coincidence that you became successful despite all you went through at Royal University? It could have gone the wrong way, couldn't it?'

There must be a perfect way of explaining God in all the grandiloquence of my stories – somehow to bring God's role closer home without the complicated narratives.

The trip to this ancient English palace would turn out to become different from many other similar relaxation trips I had embarked upon. Hampton Court Palace was one of the most magnificent royal places used by the famous King Henry VIII. One of the courtyard adornments of the palace was the Maze, a hedge spanning one-third of an acre with many turns, twists and dead ends. The Maze hedge was cut slightly above head height, having only one entrance and one exit. Therefore, this piece of architecture was famous for confusing and frustrating many visitors who would attempt to find their way through its many turns and dead ends. What a waste of time, as I hit many dead ends and kept getting lost. The puzzle of finding my way through the maze reminded me of what life could be for the youngsters I had interacted with earlier on. It also provided a picture of how my search for the ultimate ambition could have gone wrong for me. I imagined how quick the journey could be if one had a panoramic view of the Maze – then navigation would be very easy and straightforward.

Upon successful exit from The Maze, I reflected that if life and a journey to a godly ambition were the Maze, then the quickest solution would be to have a 'guidebook' with a comprehensive aerial picture. Then there would be fewer or no mistakes on the way to the proper exit point or the ultimate goal. The best routes with many advantages and fun within the complex life journey could also be maximized without missing the ultimate goal if one was to have a kind of panoramic 'guide'. That was my journey through Royal University and the many strides across Nigeria, when God had been my aerial guide. How miserable it would have been if I had insisted on my own understanding without heeding the promptings to take the most unusual routes.

The Maze was a perfect way to explain my journeys with my compassionate God. When attuned to God, His promptings (call it gut feeling or whatever), could truly be sensed and understood. God always saw the end from the very beginning, so he remained the unmistakeable best 'guide' through life.

The unforgettable work of volunteers

Sounds simple, doesn't it, but the safe keeping of the many boxes used for the mobile workshop was a big issue. The 'Roll of Honour' of Newlife Campaigns' outreach would be incomplete if certain names were omitted from it. The 10 large Pro-mobile tool chests containing equipment, various tools and spare-parts components had to be kept safe in storage at the end of each quarter's tour. The storage place had to be strategically located to aid ease of collection for the next tour. Some of my important travel documents did not necessarily have to criss-cross Nigerian deserts and forests with me, for safety reasons. They also needed strategic safe keeping whilst I was travelling within Nigeria. In the face of challenging needs, my faith in God always made me say such prayers as: 'Lord, you called me into this work as your servant; please provide me with a volunteer to assist in surmounting this or that need'. I knew I had no funding that could enable me to hire any kind of storage for the safe keeping of these items. Yet I could recollect how God had miraculously provided for these needs every step of the way.

Dammy and Chinyere (Dam-Chii) lived in Port Harcourt at the time when the Tertiary Hospital of Port Harcourt was my largest centre. I often flew Virgin Atlantic Airways directly from London Gatwick to Port Harcourt at the time. They were a lovely missionary couple who got to know about my work before I relocated to England for further education. The couple were living in the far north of Nigeria when they first came across my work. It was delightful to notice that they had been transferred to Port Harcourt by their missionary organisation, the Calvary Ministries. They quickly reconnected with me and a very strong friendship was established. The couple willingly offered to become the custodians of the workboxes at the end of every service tour when I returned to England. Damchii were the angels God sent to do the job at that period. This covered a period of over four years and I never lost any items; the chests were safely kept.

Lucy was a born neonatal nurse. She had a perfect heart

for the neonates and gave her all to ensure their survival. Then came the period when the Lagos Tertiary Hospital (LTH) became the busiest amongst all my centres. LTH's functional neonatal incubator and thermoneutral devices capacity grew. The hospital had a fleet of nearly fifty items of thermoneutral devices stationed across three sub-wards for neonatal care. Professor Akin was the CMD and he was arguably one of the best CMDs of his era, going by his love and care for the neonates. He never toyed with the maintenance of these thermoneutral systems but religiously implemented the six-monthly failure-preventive maintenance services. LTH's capacity was larger than the typical capacities of three Nigerian SCBUs combined, which necessitated the relocation of the workboxes to Lagos. Lucy's love for the neonates made her voluntarily accept the challenge of the safe keeping of the boxes. She used her influence to provide an exclusive storage space, and personally secured the room during the entire seven years of my consultancy at the hospital. Lucy was a blessing. Her services to the neonates must never go without reward, both in the present and later by God himself.

Peter (Ogene) was the best aviation expert Nigeria ever produced. He was the first to represent Africa at the World Aviation Safety Council. Ogene commanded a great deal of respect, both nationally and internationally. I knew Ogene from his early days in the city of Owerri, long before my relocation to the United Kingdom. Ogene and I served together in the Engineering Council of Owerri during those years. Ogene had a lot of character threats in common with me – no wonder we could easily tango to become great friends. Some people often referred to the two of us as 'distant twins'. Ogene grew rapidly in the aviation industry, being relocated to Lagos to head the national aviation safety offices. He understood how frustrating Nigerian public services could be, so he admired my resilience in assisting Nigeria neonates despite the fact that I so often had to fly in from the UK. Ogene would comment: 'Hippolite is an inspiration – he belonged to a top University in the world and could choose to remain comfortable there and leave Nigerians with their crazy attitudes, yet he so often tasked himself to so serve this country without minding if anyone thanked him for this or not'.

Ogene and his beautiful wife, Ngozi, were happy to offer any assistance they could to encourage me. The proximity of their residence to the Lagos airport, which I often used when flying in and out of Nigeria, provided a great help for me. Ogene's house became my local address in Nigeria, becoming my first and last point of call at the beginning and end of each consultancy mission, respectively. Ogene's family executed the function of the 'uncelebrated host' for most years of my consultancy, until Ogene's retirement from service in 2017. It would have been an incredibly difficult situation to handle if Ogene had been unwilling to play this role. He will not miss his reward because God would remember him for good for the services he did towards the preservation of neonatal lives in Nigeria.

My most valuable items and documents of great importance that were not needed further afield were all kept in safe custody at Ogene's place. I did not lose a pin in his hands. We were great friends who experienced similar difficulties in the hands of Nigerians as we tried to push the boundaries of Nigeria's 'backwardness' from our respective services. We were never short of common topics of discussion during the one or two days we had together whenever I arrived or was about to depart Nigeria. Ogene had a great sense of humour and was a very honourable man whose passion for the greatness of Nigeria was unquestionable.

Ebeleokoye was like the biblical 'Shunammite' woman. Towards the concluding years of my consultancy, matron Lucy of Lagos Tertiary Hospital retired from service. I could not find a reliable person to entrust the workboxes for safe keeping at Lagos. This was also a period when Nigerians at the centre were becoming hostile to me, perhaps due to envy. I was unwilling to take risks with my workboxes and had to look elsewhere for safe keeping within Lagos. Ebeleokoye was a lady with a golden heart. She had followed my enduring labour for Nigeria neonates for many years and aptly got to hear about the immediate need of mine. She responded: 'I am happy to use one of the free spaces at my place of residence to keep the workboxes for you'. Ebeleokoye gladly served this purpose for the remaining years of my consultancy. She was a great woman whom God provided at the right time for the neonates. As the hearts of the neonates blessed me in all my strides, so they would bless these ladies and gentlemen in the background of neonatal survival in Nigeria.

I am a decent family man. I loved my four young daughters, Jimzy, Zizi, Cherie and Matie, who needed much parental attention while growing up. My work as a parent was equally important to me. This often brought me to crossroads and difficult decisions whenever I had to abandon this aspect of my life for the quarterly four-week tour, and I was often torn apart when my daughters began to weep as I prepared to depart for Nigeria. What a sacrifice that such small children had to pay for other babies far away in the continent of Africa! The sound of their crying would ring in my ears for many days after my departure. This was not helping matters, though I would remain in constant touch to be assured everything was okay back home in England with my family.

God had blessed me with a wonderful wife who had no choice but to hold the fort whilst I was away. She wished things were different, but had to face what God's calling on my life had brought her way. Iphii was a silent but exceptional team member of Newlife Campaigns for Africa and stretched herself to the limit to ensure that I was never distracted when I was busy away in Nigeria. This was a lot of work with four energetic and demanding little daughters. I could admit that my wife Iphii was the 'hidden brick that prevented structural failure'.

Iphii needed help in England and I needed help in Nigeria – help that only God could provide using willing human tools. Bridget and her husband John, an elderly couple who lived near our residence in Hornchurch England, visited Iphii. 'It must be very difficult for you every morning, Iphii, taking your two older little girls to school whilst struggling with the twins in a double buggy,' said John. 'We have been wondering how you cope with them when Hippolite travels.'

'Yes, I am 'donating' John for the morning school drop-offs as I may still be tired and in bed,' Bridget said.

This was so amusing that it set off loud laughter from everyone present. John and Bridget were retired grandparents. John would henceforth drive to my residence every morning, park his car and walk with the children to school, a great help that could never be forgotten.

Pat Ruthven, Rebecca, Ronnie and Akwasi-Vicky were of great help to the family too. Others were my 'sister' Ikunna, my mum Nneoma-Ann who also remained in constat prayers whenever she manages to figure out that I was on 'tour', my steward at Kano hospital Mallam Chibok and my cousin Eto who assisted with my private needs in Nigeria with unrelenting loyalty, just to mention this few. These kind-hearted people numerous to mention, all members of Hornchurch Baptist Church or individual Nigerians, saw the need and willingly volunteered to fill the various gaps created by my frequent travels. They were all divinely conscripted and fulfilled great duties. Their services and actions paved the way for the saving of hundreds of thousands of African neonates. They might not know this, but each of them was God's 'angel' sent at the appointed time. The Hornchurch community, Hornchurch Baptist Church and the constituency they belonged to might not be aware of it, but the relative social and political peace my family enjoyed in this environment paved the way for the saving of thousands of African neonates. Every success I recorded in the neonatal work was theirs too.

The Reverend Minister of Hornchurch Baptist Church, the Reverend Stephen, invited me to his office. 'I have a message for you from the very last church meeting,' he said: 'The members deliberated on your passion for newborn babies around the world, especially in Africa. They talked about your unrelenting strides in creating solutions for neonates in far-away continents. They talked about your enthusiasm in your frequent updates that you willingly share with the church by notice-board posts and podium speeches. Everyone expressed the joy of being a part of this great missionary work you do.

Therefore a resolution was put forward and an overwhelming vote was cast for HBC to play a special supportive role in your great missionary work. So the church has resolved to actively remain in daily prayer for you each time you step out to Nigeria until you come back home. The church has voted for quarterly financial support to be given to you to augment your flight tickets for every quarter of the year when you travel on this mission. And every member of the church has been encouraged to volunteer the individual help each might afford for your family whenever you are away.'

I was blown away. I had not seen this coming, but was extremely excited that I was so much in the hearts of the members of HBC. I thanked the Minister and the members of HBC. However, I suggested to the church that they should consider redefining the quarterly donations to go directly towards procuring lacking medical devices which hospitals could easily acknowledge in writing: 'I believe that if the donated money was spent in this way, it would make more direct impact and be easily perceivable by the hospitals and their neonatal centres,' I said.

The church accepted this suggestion and has continued to support my medical missions in Nigeria up to the time of writing this book. I believed that the success of my great work was yet another great gift of the British people towards the global health of the international community. This was reaffirmed when I had the honour of taking the podium as one of the elected 2017 THET lecturers on the contributions of the United Kingdom towards global health, a joint conference of academia, charity, industry and the government. My great contributions might escape the UK 'radar' that monitored the country's impacts on global health owing to the fact that the work was not primarily funded by the UK; however, my work was, in no small measure, a massive achievement of the British people in literally initiating and removing a crippling problem that overwhelmed the entire nation of Nigeria.

Chuks and his amazing sacrifice

The sacrifices that many of my support workers had to face to ensure the proper delivery of our services at various times were often extreme. There were occasions when some staff risked their lives in daring circustances for these neonates.

Mr Chuks was at one time the Field Manager and was responsible for the movement of our huge work boxes. This often required him to travel the long distance from Lagos to the far north by road transport, accompanying the boxes. These journeys could continue into late hours of the next day or even into the third day due to poorly paved roads and badly maintained vehicles that could break down on the way. Mr Chuks suffered from the rare medical condition of juvenile diabetes, which continued to affect him as an adult. The management of his condition involved the observation of very strict rules of dieting and self-injection of insulin during times of diabetic crisis. He had to keep hydrated all the time and avoid starvation in order to avoid crises. On the occasion of this particular journey, the public transportation developed complicated problems that made a supposed 12-hour trip continue into the third day. The vehicle stopped at odd remote places, making it difficult for Mr Chuks to restock his water and other essentials; he later confessed his error in not taking enough stock to last well beyond the expected duration of that segment of the trip. 'This mistake was actually due to my resolve to keep a constant eye over the boxes at the motor park to ensure their careful loading into the cargo holds of the large vehicle', he said. Motor park touts are known to often 'pinch' or outrightly steal loads that are not well attended at such lawless places.

As the journey slowly progressed, Mr Chuks ran out of supplies, but he was hoping to reach the city of Lokoja, where he might visit a chemist's shop for vital medication, drinks and food. He never complained to the coach assistants, the conductors or any of his co-passengers, so no one knew his problems until he passed out with lots of strange body movements that terrified the passangers. It was only by God's divine intervention that Mr Chuks was revived as soon as they got to the city of Lokoja and was handed over to the police for interogation concerning the 'strange boxes' he was accompanying. Chuks nearly paid the ultimate price for the Nigerian neonates.

There were many people like Mr Chuks, who could never be remembered when the successes of neonatal survival in Nigeria are recounted. Chuks survived many of the subsequent trips he had to make for the neonates despite his health condition. He is celebrated in this book alongside many other senior support workers of this adventure – Chima, Jerry, Eric and Emmanuel, who at various times took extraordinary risks to ensure we had our success stories.

CHAPTER 14

A FIRST LADY TO CHAMPION THE NEONATES

✦✦✦✦✦✦✦

It was now 20 years since I had come face to face with Nigeria's neonatal mortality challenge at the Mbong Teaching Hospital. My work had since evolved into research, teaching, product and procedure development, government advocacy, product testing, validation and mass production of frugal medical devices and ideas. The work had arguably impacted the entire Nigerian nation on an unprecedented scale and literally transformed the way many Nigerian neonatologists viewed appropriate and low-cost interventions as components of lowering their extremely high neonatal mortality rate.

However, successes already achieved were yet to be exploited at scaled-up levels. It had also not been possible for me to obtain the first-ever freedom to set up what I considered an effective SCBU with appropriate and sustainable technologies for a resource-constrained country such as Nigeria. I had often been limited by what an individual Chief Medical Director had chosen to do or the extent to go for the neonatal ward. I was often frustrated when they jettisoned my ideas for rather more expensive approaches which I already knew would fail. I had a mental picture of what the ideal SCBU in Nigeria should look like, but never had the opportunity or free hand to actualize this, and by so doing, enable other hospitals to observe the difference and perhaps copy it. Sadly, after 20-odd years I had given up of this ever coming to pass.

Princess Nikky, the Princess Royale of Wazobialand, was no doubt the African golden lady of the era. She championed the campaign against breast and prostate cancer in African and had a very strong working collaboration with the African First Ladies Forum (AFLAF). The AFLAF was the umbrella forum that brought the wives and spouses of the presidents, prime ministers and heads of states of African countries together to discuss issues of common interest. The Princess Royale was also the Secretary General of the African Union Women Assembly, headquartered at the AU House Addis Ababa, Ethiopia. The Princess Royale Cancer Organisation assisted in the strengthening and sustainability of the AFLAF, transforming this into an influential and reputable organisation in Africa.

Being a mother herself, the Wazobialand Princess Royale was sympathetic to the plight of the poor dying neonates in Africa and often wished she could help. During one of her interviews on breast cancer in Africa, the Princess was emotionally upset about the way Africa was riddled with so many problems to solve, including high neonatal mortality across the continent. She was unaware of the work I was doing in the African nation of Nigeria. The Princess was thrilled to hear one of the interviewers talk about the visions and exploits of one Professor Hippolite in Nigeria. She did not hesitate, afterwards, to contact me to know more about my work. She consequently shared the gathered information with the executive of the AFLAF, leading to my invitation to address African First Ladies at the AU House in Addis Ababa, Ethiopia, during one of their summer summits.

The meeting was scheduled for the first week in August. I had been busy with many international engagements during the year, including one that ended in Paris, France during the last week of July. I was visibly exhausted from travelling and needed to return home to England for a good rest. I loved the idea of speaking to the African First Ladies, but I wished the summit was not scheduled so early in August.

On the last day of the France meeting, I was seriously worried that I would not attend the Ethiopian meeting and contemplated sending an email to notify the African princess and the AFLAF that I would not be coming. I walked to a vacant seat, sat down and pulled out my laptop to send the email.

'Hello, good afternoon,' greeted a gentleman on the adjacent seat.

'Hi, nice to meet you. I am Hippolite.'

I shook his hand, intending to quickly return to my computer, but the man would not let go of my hand. 'I really enjoyed your powerful speech during the last session and wish more black men could make it to the world stage and be as brave as you are,' he said. 'I am Mr Kumbala. I come from Ethiopia and work for the World Health Organisation there.'

'Thank you for the compliments, nice to hear you are from Ethiopia,' I said.

'Have you ever been to Ethiopia?' asked Mr Kumbala.

'No. I am about to cancel an invitation to go there for the first time next week,' I replied.

Mr Kumbala was quite a chatty man and almost distracted me from the quick email I wanted to send. I told him why I had been planning on going to Ethiopia, and Mr Kumbala got emotional and passionately pleaded that my mission to Ethiopia was such an important one that it should not be aborted. It was as though he had been divinely sent to prevail on me to reconsider what I was about to do. He provided me with statistics for dying African neonates – situations I already knew – insisting that a bold and accomplished professional like me needed to urgently speak to African first ladies about this. He explained how much his country would benefit from such a speech from me.

'You have almost persuaded me to forget my tiredness for the sake of the neonates,' I said, with a smile on my face. Another handshake and it was time for the next session at the Paris conference. I could not send the email, but Mr Kumbala's words continued to reverberate in my mind as I headed for my hotel room at the end of the last session of the conference.

I finally decided to make the Ethiopian meeting, but I had only three days to fly back to England, get ready and proceed on the African journey.

The following week, I was in Addis Ababa, Ethiopia, for the First Ladies Forum summit. The cocktail reception event at the classy Radisson Blu Hotel was full of gorgeously-dressed Africans in their brilliant colours. The food and drink was fantastic. A lot of people were meeting for the first time and introducing themselves to one another. Old friends could be seen laughing and catching up with discussions whilst they sipped their drinks, standing around tables filled with various items of food to nibble. Participants had come from all over Africa, in addition to invited guests from around the world. I was soaking up the atmosphere too as I sipped my glass of wine.

Suddenly, there was a gentle tap on my shoulder. I turned around to find myself being offered a handshake. 'Hello, I am Ahmed Abu from Nigeria,' said the gentleman. 'Are you the professor from the Royal University London who is due to speak at the conference tomorrow?'

'Yes I am,' I replied.

'I am part of the team from Nigeria. We were reading and discussing your profile as one member of my team drew our attention to it. You've had some impressive achievements in your career. I am glad to finally meet you in person,' said Ahmed, and with another handshake, he walked away.

Ahmed returned to me before the end of the evening, accompanied by a lady delegate from his Nigerian team. They had a special request for me: 'Sir,' she said, 'I have been sent by the leader of the Nigerian delegation, Her Excellency Amina the First Lady of Kainji State of Nigeria, to request a chat with you.'

I accepted the proposal to meet with the Most Excellent

Amina that same evening – a meeting that lasted only six minutes, involving a quick summary of my African research and work among Nigerian neonates. Amina was awed, amazed and excited as I gave my three-minute summary. She beamed at me as I concluded by saying: 'Ma'am, you could hear more, I hope, during my speech tomorrow'.

Amina responded, 'I am glad to hear you hold Nigerian citizenship as well. I am a consultant gynaecologist by profession. I would be pleased if you can agree for us to have a more detailed meeting before the end of the conference'.

'Sure, it will be my pleasure,' I said as I bowed and walked away.

Within 15 minutes of departing from The Most Excellent Amina, Ahmed, her protocol officer, approached me again to discuss scheduling two more separate meetings for discussions with his First Lady. I sensed the unusual seriousness and interest from this lady, so I determined to keep these appointments and made up my mind to offer the best advice possible.

The time finally arrived and Her Excellency began: 'I am passionately seeking the best possible ways of doing something substantial for the maternal and neonatal health of my state in Nigeria. I knew this would require some exceptional and unique input from a well-experienced professional. I have been able to set things rolling at a level based on the best advice and assistance I have been able to access so far in my country. We have completed a facility building, and scheduled to open it by next month, September. However, I somehow feel that what we have in place is not exactly to the standard I have in mind for the Centre. What we have on the ground is not very different from the failed methodologies that existed in tertiary hospitals in the past, at least to the best of my knowledge. I have the urge in my heart to do something better, but I don't know what I should do differently.'

I stared at the First Lady, relishing the passion for the neonatal cause she was expressing. I knew that The Most Excellent Amina was a gynaecologist and also the wife of a politician; however, I could not believe the passion and intensity with which she was delivering her report. Never in my twenty years of concerted efforts in Nigeria had I heard any politician speak with such passion for the neonates. I was blown away, and almost could not believe what the First Lady was saying. Was this woman attempting to impress me? Was she just another garrulous person from the Nigerian political class trying to impress me? She might not be aware how much of Nigeria I knew or how easily I could investigate her authenticity.

Amina continued: 'How I wish you could have a look at what we have got at Hadeja, Kainji state capital city, and advise us before we open the facility for services. Having read about you and your vast experience, I have the strong feeling you would be of great help to us.'

'I know so much about Nigeria and its neonatal needs, and I am impressed with your vision to establish an exceptional neonatal centre like no other in Nigeria,' I replied. 'I have big ideas about what an exceptional, appropriate, sustainable and low-cost SCBU in a typical African country should look like. However, I am not sure this could be what you have in mind. In any case, I must tell you that I am interested in being a part of some neonatal innovations, but I will be unable to come to Nigeria until October'.

The First Lady's eyes lit up. 'Quite frankly, Prof, I can call Nigeria right away to ask them to suspend plans for the opening of the facility if you promise to come to us in October,' she said.

After the Addis Ababa conference, I had a couple of telephone updates and discussions with the First Lady and finally set a date for my maiden visit. I had done a lot of research and was impressed with her work, and I was determined in my heart to offer her the best possible assistance within the limits of her resources.

I flew to Abuja airport and completed the remaining three-hour journey by road in the company of one of my Nigerian junior registrars, Dr Temilade. The federal highway and roads between Abuja and Hadeja were horribly bumpy due to potholes that dotted almost the entire length. The journey was hence a very stressful one for me, and I was glad when we arrived safely. The First Lady's chief protocol officer, Ahmed, was waiting for me at the main arched gate of the city of Hadeja and led me to the new facility, where the First Lady was already awaiting my arrival.

I had no idea of the surprises that awaited me as Ahmed led me upstairs to the conference room of the new neonatal hospital. I had expected to see the First Lady in the room with, perhaps, one or two aides. As we approached the door, Ahmed pointed at a seat in a small seating area and said: 'Prof, please have a seat and I will be with you shortly'. He went inside the conference room and shut the door behind him. He returned after a couple of minutes and said, 'Sir, could you please come with me?' Unbelievable!

The room was packed full of people neatly dressed in

different colourful traditional office attires. They were sitting on well-arranged chairs round the conference room table. Almost 100 pairs of eyes instantly fixed on me as I stepped in with the young doctor that accompanied me. At the executive end of the Boardroom Table sat Her Excellency Amina the First Lady, smiling as she planted her lovely eyes on me. Her excitement was unmistakable. I had won a place in her heart for remaining true to my promises to visit. 'This must be a man of integrity,' the look in her eyes seemed to be saying.

Unknown to me, the First Lady had got down to work as soon as she returned from the Addis Ababa meeting. She had detailed her aides to do more research into Professor Hippolite of the Royal University London. The result of the search was overwhelming to her office staff, one reporting back: 'Your Excellency, the current search has shown that we really knew very little about the numerous quiet achievements of this Professor'. She was thrilled that a man of such global prowess could be as simple as the figure she had met at the Ethiopian meeting, and felt really glad that I had accepted her invitation without much hesitation. She had shared her discoveries with her husband, His Excellency the Governor, and asked his approval for the First Lady to use her advocacy services to foster a collaboration that could boost the survival rate of neonates in their state. Her husband pledged his support, and so Amina, like an ancient warrior, began her plans for an overwhelming reception for me. In the 20 years of my work in Nigeria, I had never been received by such a welcome party in any of the states or tertiary hospitals of Nigeria. I had already concluded that Nigerians were people who rarely appreciated good gestures, even when these had been done sacrificially as with the numerous cases in my risky work across Nigeria. The Most Excellent Amina had stepped in to change all that without even knowing what she had done. She had circulated information round all senior health workers in her vast state, one of the largest Nigerian states by land mass, notifying them of the visit. From across the state, these senior health officers and the State Commissioner for Health had assembled together for this grand reception.

Amina formally introduced me and in turn introduced her top senior staff of the Ministry of Health. I was so humbled by the First Lady's gesture, more especially when she presented a gift to me – a beautifully woven official regalia with the symbol of her state on it, a wonderful memento indeed.

There were a couple of short speeches before the top senior officers conducted me and the First Lady round the new neonatal hospital building for my observation and comments. I made my notes, assisted by my student doctor, Dr Temilade, as we moved from one section of the building to the other. There were questions, answers and counter questions as I tried to explain the very visible mistakes already made, thereby preparing the minds of the officers for what could shortly follow in my comprehensive assessment report. It was an exhaustive exercise but very convincing and satisfying to all the medical seniors who joined in the hospital round.

I repeated my promise to assist them in making the neonatal hospital the best of its kind in Nigeria if they were happy with my proposals, which would soon follow. Everyone was excited by my visit, and people were seen expressing their thanks to the First Lady because of my obvious vast experience in my various comments during the round. They could not wait to see things put in motion to actualise the ambitious ideas being proposed to them. There were, of course, a lot of attendees who had never heard of me until now. Dr Temilade overheard different groups discussing the passion and intelligence in my speeches and advice. Dr Temilade also noted that some wondered if such a talented intellectual and great global figure was actually a Nigerian, as the country had not been able to maximise the assistance I could offer at the national level. One said: 'What thrills me most is his humility; I will see how far we could go with him.'

At the end of the tour of the facility, the last part of the visit began. This was another meeting in the boardroom. Amina chaired this meeting and the attendance was limited to the Commissioner of Health, the Permanent Secretary and the Directors of the Ministry of Health. Dr Temilade sat next to me as my assistant and team member. Amina thanked me for keeping to my promise of coming to Nigeria to visit her state. She expressed her delight that I had passed what she referred to as 'the first test of this collaboration'. She said: 'Prof, it is so common these days for people to try to impress me by making empty promises, especially people from far-away countries, so your visit alone has given me great joy, and I know you must have noticed that it is not just I but the majority of the people who came to welcome you. So, once again you are very welcome to our state'.

She allowed more reactions from the Commissioner, the Permanent Secretary and two other Directors of the Ministry of Health, all of them commenting on their impressions from what I had said during the facility round. They spoke of their excitement about the project, and also their worries and the potential difficulties that could be encountered based on some of the proposals for alterations, devices and staff training that I had already mentioned. Dr Amina's summarizing speech was rather long as she tried to clearly explain that the collaboration had already started in her mind and that she would, in her capacity, ensure that the collaboration turned out to be one that could make everyone proud. She maintained that funding might be an issue, but they would not let go of me as I possessed the necessary experience the state could tap into to actualise this dream.

Looking round the table again and leaning forward, Amina said: 'Ladies and gentlemen, you have seen and heard from the man himself and I am sure you can see why I never gave up in my drive to bring him here'. And looking at me, she said: 'We can appreciate the benefits that could be derived from your ideas of appropriate devices and layout you have shared with us. These all sound great, but as you may notice from the worries expressed by other speakers, the scale of this project might involve huge amounts of money that we might be unable to fund. I am sure these worries stem from previous experiences of projects of similar scales'.

I responded: 'Your Excellency, ladies and gentlemen: believe me, even if we do not go ahead to collaborate, the gesture I have received so far will continue to be relished in my heart. However, I must promise you that your passion to help these poor neonates alone can throw up surprises you are not expecting. Your Excellency, I am going to make an unusual request, of a type I am sure is not common in Nigeria.'

'Please go ahead,' responded the First Lady.

'Irrespective of how inadequate your budget might be, we

could still work out a great deal for the neonates. I do not know how much the Governor wishes to spend, but you need to think about entrusting this money to my hands and I will deliver a result that will surprise you. I am aware of stories of people running away with public funds. This is common in this country, but you might need to consider taking the risk of trusting me, because then you can expect results without delays. Can you give me one week to prepare my work plan: facility layout, training and devices in a budget proposal for you to study? I will use a scalable technique that can easily expand or shrink facility capacity based on the available funding, irrespective of the size. We could set up a functional centre with expansion allowance to grow to full capacity whenever more funds become available. I am primarily going to use your centre to display my professional artistry in its finest details, though within the limits of your funding ability. I plan to deploy the best of my frugal medical devices and procedures to put up a centre of excellence here. If you are happy with my request, then we have a deal.'

As I concluded my speech, I looked at the faces of all the people sitting round the table and saw expressions of reassurance.

'Great, I think you have summed it up, Prof. We have a deal then,' said the First Lady. She thanked all the people in the room for coming and closed the meeting. I was so happy about all that had happened. I cherished the respect and honour from this highly-placed but humble woman. As we rose from our seats, I could confidently say that I had just experienced my highest state honour in my 20 years of sacrificial services to the Nigerian people. But how wrong I was. The First Lady turned to me and said: 'By the way Prof, there is one more item on the agenda before you depart back to Abuja – a state banquet in your honour to be hosted by me. My entourage is waiting for us outside to drive us to the State House where this banquet has been arranged. I hope you don't mind?'

I was astonished, and couldn't believe what I just heard. 'Sure, Your Excellency, it's an honour. Thank you,' I responded, as we all dispersed and headed for the State House.

The beauty of Amina's heart was clearly portrayed in her charming personality. She was one of those rare gems of womanhood, motherhood and professional integrity. She loved her profession as a gynaecologist and obstetric surgeon, but this did not limit her zeal to use her privileged position to provide help for the poor. In all my experiences in the field, I could say confidently that I had never met any woman as passionate for the survival of the neonate as Amina. Could her character represent the assistance the Nigerian neonates required to survive? Her persistent drive in this project would be essential in a country where the civil servants were the 'caterpillars' that destroyed the nation and devoured her resources.

I knew a lot about how civil servants destroy projects as they connive with dubious contractors to divide and share money meant for them. Kainji State could pull pleasant surprises in presenting a different set of Ministry of Health civil servants in terms of character; after all God had used the emergence of Amina to prove to me that some 'golden hearts' could still be found among the political class. Knowing this, however, I must apply caution to find a way of ensuring that any funding money was maximized to bring to reality an enviable neonatal centre for this state.

The third quarter medical mission was progressing very well. My team was out working at the hospitals on the mission schedule. Mr Chuks, my most senior technical assistant (the Field Manager, FM) would keep my mobile phone whilst at work. This enabled us to avoid the frequent distractions from people calling me for unimportant reasons. The FM answered my calls, identified callers and only passed the phone to me if the call required my immediate input.

Mr Chuks stepped forward: 'Excuse me Prof, you have a call from the First Lady,' he said. I took the phone. 'A very good afternoon, Your Excellency; can I be of any help?'

'Thank you Prof for all the documents you have been sending to us in answer to our various requests all along. I really appreciate them,' she said. 'All the relevant officers of the Ministry of Health have gone through your list – the alterations to be done in the building, the staff training aspect and the medical devices to be deployed. Everyone seems to worry about the cost implications – these might involve huge sums of money. We are also wondering if some of the items could wait until the hospital has been opened for work. The cost of staff training for the first batch of doctors and nurses is known. The Ministry of Health has also quantified the cost of building alterations based on your new designs. Our fear is that not much money would be left for the long list of the medical devices in the document you sent. The Governor is making available a specific amount of money for this project and might not be willing to accept requests for additional funding. I felt I should discuss this with you.'

Amina was quite exhaustive in detailing the dilemma. She wished there were no obstacles against the progress of the project; however, she preferred not to be over presumptuous in the management of the meagre funding.

I listened attentively and in response, I said: 'We compulsorily need the stated number of doctors and nurses to be available and specially trained ahead of the opening of the Centre – this one is not negotiable. The management of Abuja University Hospital has accepted my request regarding the intended training of Hadeja SCBU staff using AUH facilities. Hence, we have started planning for six months 'residential' training of the Hadeja staff at Abuja hospital. Your Excellency, there is only one more piece of help I can offer – tell me the exact amount of money the Governor is prepared to spend on the devices, commit this to my hands and I will make it to go round in the best way possible. I know that it might not be easy to do this due to civil service rules and the so-called 'due process' agenda in Nigeria civil service; however, I do not have any other way of assisting. I guess in order to avoid awarding contracts to suppliers that might be unable to provide the kind of devices I wish to use, the Ministry of Health might be better off allowing me to personally supervise the supply of the devices I need'.

'Okay Prof, I will deliver this message to the directors at the Ministry of Health during our next meeting scheduled for tomorrow. Everyone thinks that the state is lucky that both of us seem to understand each other; so they rely on my ability to convince you to offer unconventional help to the State. Prof, I really appreciate all your effort and help so far. Thank you,' she concluded.

The Most Excellent Amina was now overworking all her team members to ensure that all the necessary executive approvals were given quickly enough to enable me to commence work on the project before the end of my current consultancy visit in Nigeria.

I began to get calls from other senior directors of the Ministry of Health – Permanent Secretary, Director of Works and Planning, Director Statistics, Executive Medical Director, Director of Finance, etc. – each trying to obtain clarification for their own aspects of work involved in the project. Everyone was eager to ensure that the project did not fail from his own end. I had never experienced such efficiency in a Nigerian civil service system in the twenty years of my neonatal outreach in Nigeria. This was a pleasant surprise indeed! Each of the directors spoke with respect and a thankful attitude to my generosity and patriotism. I had never felt so appreciated.

The Permanent Secretary, Dr Mohammed (Makus), called: 'Prof, I must say how greatly we are encouraged, challenged and motivated by your strength of purpose and drive for these achievements. I am accustomed to doing things differently to achieve results even from my last posting as the head of a specialist hospital in the State. This is the reason some immoral people don't like my style and are doing all they can to eliminate me, but they won't succeed. I am happy you have come to execute this extraordinary project in the Ministry while I am the Permanent Secretary of Health in our state. My promise to you is that I will do everything in my power to ensure that this project is delivered exactly how you wish it done. We are all excited, including the Honourable Commissioner, that someone of your status has been brought into this project. The success of this project will be another big plus on our respective CVs. We are currently working on all the papers that have been submitted by the various Directors and you will be contacted as quickly as possible for your next course of action, sir.'

Wow! Knowing what happens in the Nigerian civil service, I could not believe that a Permanent Secretary had just called with this sort of passion and promise of commitment for the successful completion of a project he had not been bribed for. This civil servant had not asked for his 'cuts' or how much would be diverted into his private pocket. There had been no funny 'body language' as I was accustomed to observing in situations like this. In all these calls, I had taken all the promises with a pinch of salt until the funds had been released.

Another two days passed and another phone call came through, this time from the Director of Planning: 'We have been holding meetings to review the list you submitted, sir. We now have directives from Mr Governor in which we have been notified that approval for the project funds has been given. Unfortunately, we won't be having a lot of money left after the costs of the staff residential training programme at Abuja and the cost of your re-designed building reconstructions and alterations has all been taken out. Everyone is keen to see this project succeed, so we are ready to assist in any way possible, sir. We have agreed that all tenders for the supply of medical devices listed in your document would be passed through you. We want you to select the most convincing contractors that could deliver what you need for the centre. There are still some of the devices you listed that have not been tendered for; perhaps these devices are not readily available in Nigeria. Moreover we observed that contractors have quoted huge amounts of money for the rest of the devices, so that the funding left for this cannot even go one third of the way.'

'We were also wondering if you could kindly agree to handle the sourcing of these items in the best and most cost-effective manner, as you earlier suggested. We are going to reconvene later in the day and I am expected to return with any guidance from you, sir.'

In response, I said: 'Thank you Director for the great job you are doing. I am glad that all of you are committed to the success of this project. I am prepared to go the extra mile if need be to assist. Hence, I am happy to take up the challenge of contacting capable companies or individuals – from within and outside Nigeria – to negotiate deals for urgent delivery of the devices at the most efficient costs. This is my promise. I am aware of the civil service rules that might constrain you from the use of the released funds for upfront payment of the devices. However, I am basically an academic and not necessarily a businessman; hence, I will require this money to be given to me upfront so it is to hand for prompt settlement with the companies willing to make deals with me.'

'This is the ugly bit,' said the Director. 'We know the bottleneck lies with this limitation that you are already aware of. I will also make your position on this matter known to the rest of the Directors during the meeting. Thank you for your time, sir.'

I remained a highly respected visiting professor and consultant at the Special Care Baby Unit of the Abuja University Hospital. The management of the hospital held me in the highest esteem and treated my suggestions with the greatest respect. I designed a six-month residential training programme covering all aspects of neonatal care for the Hadeja take-off clinical and nursing staff to be hosted in the Paediatrics Department of AUH. Resource persons for the training were drawn from the rich staff team and members of my research group in the special care baby unit of AUH.

I finally submitted my teaching and training programme to the management of AUH and encouraged them to carefully negotiate training facility and administrative costs with the Ministry of Health of Kainji State. I cleverly linked the two organisations together and brokered their deal for collaboration. With the MoU signed between Kainji State Ministry of Health and AUH, I was set to go. The commencement date for the arriving trainees was set. This promptly kicked off as scheduled.

The building and interior alteration work at the Hadeja Neonatal Hospital started at the same time that trainees arrived in Abuja to commence studies. This was planned to ensure quick completion in readiness for the returning trainees six months later and hence the commissioning of the facility. All the devices intended for installation were expected to be sourced, delivered and installed within this time period too. It was thrilling for me as I carefully observed the project taking off as planned without the well-known Nigerian civil servants' greed and demands for bribes.

For the Permanent Secretary, it was all hands on deck as he went all out motivating all his directors and encouraging them to show a good account of themselves. Time was beginning to run out on the ordering of the necessary devices as set out in my working document. The Permanent Secretary and his directors must find a way of moving this aspect forward. The PS himself would not take chances with some unreliable equipment suppliers in Nigeria. He was nearing conclusion with his directors to take a dive into his most frightening risk ever.

A call came through from the Permanent Secretary: 'Prof, we are almost stranded, as we are not convinced that we can risk putting our hope in our local suppliers for the indicated medical devices. I may have to take the risk of my life, risking my position and job, in order to move this project forward. By civil service rules, I will be held responsible if things go wrong with the steps I have decided to take now. I have carefully observed you for as long as we have come in contact and I have the confidence that you are a God-fearing man, so I am happy to take this risk of trusting you. Shortly after this call, the Director of Planning will be sending you an official request for a local bank account number to which we can transfer the approved funding for the devices. We have all agreed to take this step together as everyone is at peace with you and the personality you have displayed so far. Congratulations Prof for this; nowadays in Nigeria, there are more bad people than good, so no one takes this kind of risk for anyone, except of course partners in crime. Please don't get me wrong. We had silent opposition from a few people, though. They argued that it was not fair to hand the entire money over to one person to manage instead of distributing the supply job through the Ministry's network of suppliers. It is understandable, because this is what they have been used to doing in the past, but the current project is one that I am not comfortable to put in the hands of our local suppliers. Many of the directors share the same view, so we had no difficulty voting in favour of committing everything to you. We are all proud of the fact that you are such a global figure and also a Nigerian. Please do not hesitate to keep me posted in case of any difficulties. I will also appreciate it if you could send us a written acknowledgement for any payments you receive.'

I was glad the Hadeja team had finally taken this decision. The team was expecting the small amount left for medical devices which had been transferred to me to achieve the procurement of up to half the items listed in the working document. I, however, was determined to give them a pleasant surprise by doing everything in my power to acquire all the devices with the meagre funding presented. I had some plans for how to go about this.

The Permanent Secretary, Dr Makus, acted exactly as promised. My Newlife Campaigns for Africa bank account got credited with the entire money released for the supply and installation of the neonatal devices for the Centre. What a surprise! I had to modify my theory about Nigerian civil servants. They might not all be the 'caterpillars' that devoured the nation. Dr Makus has shown himself to be a completely different breed of civil servant. I made up my mind to repay his honesty by showing him how such a small amount of money could be used to fund the entire list of devices – though it would be a challenge.

I returned to England and got to work. I made contacts with manufacturers and suppliers within the UK and European Union soliciting assistance to enable me to execute a 'charitable work for African neonates'. This yielded a lot of positive results in terms of discounts and free deliveries to Nigeria or the UK. I kept my eyes on the available funds to maximise their potential reach. I received a lot of discounts which enabled me secure all the items in the list, while leaving me with some money to commit to other devices that had been left out due to the poor funding.

With all items on the list ticked, I had to work towards transferring the funds in my Naira-denominated account in Nigeria to my United Kingdom Nat West Bank account to enable me make payments to all the companies and suppliers that had promised to assist me. None of these companies agreed to ship their products to Nigeria or my local address in England without 100% payment of the costs in advance. I was aware of the stringent UK rules and regulations on money laundering. I had to apply caution to avoid problems. I had never operated a business account in the United Kingdom, and had no plans to open one, since the present project was the first of its kind, and probably a one-off in my 20 years of neonatal charity in Nigeria.

I contacted my manager at the Nigerian Diamond Bank for help, but found that the bank was not willing to apply the official exchange rate to transfer the funds. This would mean a huge loss of value, thereby limiting my ability to secure all the negotiated items of medical devices. I discovered that the bank officials used the allocated foreign exchange from the Nigerian Central Bank to enrich themselves. They hawked this to 'black market' operators, and later bought it back to be sold to people like me at higher cost. This was a disgusting and disturbing revelation that I could not stand. I decided to leave the Diamond Bank alone after it refused to show any sympathy for the dying neonates: 'Diamond Bank's hard-heartedness is another reason why Nigerian neonates have died,' I said to the Manager and hung up the phone, never to call again on this matter. It was so surprising that highly-educated Nigerians like these bankers were not bothered that their country was bedevilled with such a high neonatal mortality rate. 'God forbid a nation where the pursuit of money is more important than human life,' I would say aloud as the thoughts of all these disturbed me.

CHAPTER 15

STRANGLED BY A BANK'S RED TAPE

✦✦✦✦✦✦✦

I worried about the fund transfer problem for some days without any solution in sight. Finally I resolved to move forward. There was no room for failure, so I would have to find other methods. I made several calls for advice. One good piece of advice came from a British travel agency I had used in the past, a private company owned by a Nigerian-born British man. The Director, Mr Suratu, was shocked to hear about the high mortality statistics of Nigerian neonates when I presented the case to him. He was sympathetic and promised to help me. Mr Suratu's company had naira bank accounts with the Nigerian Diamond Bank, so he was happy to arrange for instalment payments of British sterling into my UK bank account provided I was prepared to refund the naira equivalent into his Diamond Bank account in Nigeria. The most interesting aspect was that Mr Suratu would exchange the funds at official rates prevailing on the days his account was credited in Nigeria. This promise sounded great to me. However, there was a problem. The United Kingdom anti-money laundering systems could easily misunderstand large payments into my account, thereby triggering a security alert.

I decided to contact NatWest Bank first to explore the possibility of obtaining approval to allow me to use my account for this important project. During the discussion with the bank's customer services officer, Mr Oleg, I clearly informed him about my twenty years of charitable services in Nigeria and all the circumstances leading to this peculiar project: 'I am fully aware of the anti-money laundering laws in the United Kingdom and must seek for your permission and approval before using my account to do this work of mercy,' I said.

The NatWest bank staff collected all the necessary account details, and asked me to send my Diamond Bank account statement from which these transfers would be initiated. He particularly wished to see payments into this account from the Ministry of Health Hadeja to authenticate my story. All this was done as requested, and the NatWest bank officer told me that I could go ahead with the plan.

Mr Suratu, the travel agent, was a trustworthy gentleman. He delivered his promises and credited my NatWest bank account at the best exchange rates. I did not hesitate to reimburse his Nigerian naira account as agreed. The transaction between

Suratu and me was gentlemanly until the full amount was transferred, which was a great relief for me. I was so thankful to God.

Several payments were made to a number of UK and European companies and suppliers from my NatWest account. All the organisations lived up to their promises of discounts or free deliveries. Some shipped their items straight to Nigeria, while others shipped to my UK residential address.

I obtained the best respiratory-support devices and phototherapy systems from a Vietnamese company, MTTS Asia. The sum of 15,000 US dollars had to be transferred to them before the dispatch of the items to Nigeria. I made a walk-in appointment to effect the transfer over the counter at the NatWest branch in Romford, United Kingdom. I had expected this to be without any hitch until the cashier said: 'hang on a minute; it looks like payment has been denied and a red alert triggered on my computer. I'm sorry but this cannot be completed and your account has been shut down.'

'Why? What do you mean?' I asked.

'I can see that there have been many transactions in and out of this account recently. I am afraid this account is now frozen and you will not be able to operate it again until you have been contacted by one of our staff. Expect a call from us or a letter in the post in this regard. I am so sorry,' said the NatWest branch supervisor.

I thought it was a joke until I left the bank and tried to connect to my online banking but was refused access to my account. I waited for three days, but there was no phone call or letter from NatWest bank. I made attempts to speak to someone at NatWest, but none had any information as to what had gone wrong and why my account was frozen.

After two weeks without any information, I went to my NatWest South Kensington branch and had a chat with the manager. I explained all I could about my Nigerian project, the neonatal mercy work, my initial discussions and approval from NatWest bank. I asked why NatWest had misled me in the first place by approving the use of this account to execute the project. I wanted to know why my account was frozen. I wanted to know how long the NatWest investigation on my account would last, and above all I wanted my branch manager to confirm if I was directly being investigated as a criminal or not.

Unfortunately I received no answers to these questions, except that I was told that the problem was not necessarily directed at me personally. I was struck dumb when the manager revealed that the investigation could take up to six months to conclude, during which I would have no access to my account or the Hadeja funds in it.

I was devastated. I explained again to the manager that the money in the account was not mine: 'I am only a university researcher passionate to help some dying babies in Africa. The money came from a meagre funding by poor people who dared to care about these dying infants. Please don't let NatWest be among the murderers of innocent babies in Africa, please, please,' I pleaded with the manager. 'The poor Africans trusted me and committed their little money in my care because they believed I would not dupe them. They are expecting me to return with their medical devices within the next few weeks.

Please don't let me go to them with 'hard-to-believe' stories of their money being frozen in the United Kingdom!'

The heartless NatWest manager made fruitless calls to unknown distant faceless security officers. I finally announced to the embattled manager that I was not going to leave the banking hall until I received proper answers or was handed over to the police. This move initially looked like a joke to the banking staff, until it was time for the bank to close for work. I was not prepared to leave the building. Every plea from the bank staff and the manager fell on deaf ears. I was determined even to struggle with the police so as to create a public scene.

After long hours of unsuccessful attempts to persuade me to leave the bank, the manager threatened to call the police. 'Please be quick as this is what I have been waiting for,' I angrily replied. The manager consulted with a few other staff, made other calls and returned to me to plead: 'You see, I do really appreciate your frustrations and I wish it was in my power to resolve this matter. I can promise you that I do not have any clue or answer to any of your questions. If I did, I would not hesitate to give it. I also know that continuing to stay here even through this night would not change the situation. You will only be creating problems for the two of us, sadly. So I beg you to leave the bank and I promise to personally give this another chase tomorrow. However, I am not making any promises that my report will influence the ongoing investigation.'

There had been some angry scenes in the banking hall since my arrival. I decided to leave, even though I had had no answers to my questions. What would be the fate of the Hadeja neonatal project and the money committed into my hands? I had been waiting for the bank for eight weeks, and still had no clue. I had not told Nigeria about the ordeal I had been going through. I was well aware of the disbelief such a story would generate. I would not put my reputation to ridicule in Nigeria – I was determined that this problem would never reach the ears of Nigerians until the project was fully delivered with no excuses. The white supremacist's witch-hunt such as NatWest Bank had displayed was another reason why African and Nigerian neonates died. I would have to find a new way of putting my energy back into the project to deliver this at the set time. But how might the project be put back on course? I looked towards my numerous friends and sympathizers for help.

I first convinced myself that NatWest could never freeze the Hadeja money forever. They could only frustrate me by delaying my access to the funds for a time. I was not going to give up. I was sure that I had done nothing wrong; hence, NatWest could do either of two things at the end: let me resume control of the funds or return the money to the Kainji state account in Nigeria. If I could find someone to borrow from, I could refund them as soon as NatWest allowed me to regain access to my funds.

I ruled out soliciting for money from any of my numerous United Kingdom mission supporters. This was because I was not sure of the extent the devil was using NatWest Bank to attack the poor tiny Nigerian neonates. They could be monitoring any payments with my name going out of the United Kingdom. There was no room for a second disaster!

I had only one set of friends to turn to – those in the USA. I preferred to approach some long-time friends within my Christian Fellowship organisation – the NIFESAF. My reputation and integrity had been impeccable and unquestionable. My services, love and philanthropy within the brotherhood of the Fellowship had been phenomenal. I would only have to approach a few well-to-do members of this Fellowship to raise the needed funds and pay MTTS-Asia directly from the USA. I was not the kind of figure in this Fellowship to be denied my cry for help; at least that was my impression at the time. I had sacrificially borne the burden of this fellowship for many years in the past, both to individual members and the fellowship as an institution. I never gave any thought to failure for help from the members of NIFESAF at my difficult time.

But I was wrong. People do not realise how lonely they really are until they find themselves stranded. Yes, the philanthropist and a long-time helper of his Christian friends was finally stranded, and crying out for help that fell on deaf ears. Those I asked to help raise the money for my problem provided me with well-crafted excuses. The bottom line was that these people failed me when the neonates and I needed them most. I had ever enjoyed being the giver and not the receiver by all standards and as much as I could remember in my life or in the history of my membership of this Christian organisation. I thought I would readily be treated as I had treated many others, but it was not so this time. This group with their professions of 'brotherly love' had revealed their true colours towards me. I loved with all my heart, but my smart friends had shown me that love could be with the corner of the heart only.

The fact is that humans can throw ugly surprises with unacceptable excuses. However, God can choose to use anyone at any time to achieve His purposes. My motives were heaven ordained, so I knew that God would not leave me stranded for too long or allow my reputation to be scorned in Nigeria, and so it was. Help came from elsewhere, and God made a way for me where there seemed to be none. The correct amount of money was obtained from another source outside my Christian friends. A true sympathizer came to my rescue. The full amount was wired through to the MTTS Asia account in Hong Kong, and the goods were paid for in full – hallelujah!

MTTS Asia promptly delivered the devices to Nigeria and I was back on course, racing towards the project completion deadline without any more pressure or fear of failure.

The staff training courses at the AUH Abuja went as planned. The construction and alteration work of the hospital building were completed. All devices were delivered, assembled and installed in readiness for the commissioning day. Everyone at Hadeja Ministry of Health was happy to see the quality and quantity of the medical devices the meagre funding achieved. There was unreserved appreciation and thanksgiving for my excellent display of efficiency pouring in from the Directors of the Ministry of Health. The Most Excellent Amina was ecstatic with the extent of the success scored. She happily delivered the special appreciation of the State Governor to me. The Neonatal Hospital was turned into an excellent facility which I assessed as second to none in Nigeria in terms of the availability and quality of medical technology. During the commissioning of the facility no one ever challenged my claim that the new Hadeja Special Care Baby Unit stood out amongst Nigeria's tertiary centres. This was an ambitious statement to make; however, I had been everywhere in Nigeria doing this neonatal work. I had superior information and could quickly make such assessments and conclusions. The Hadeja people were happy with what they got from this project, but at the same time, they took my claim with a pinch of salt.

I concluded my work and handed over the centre to the hands of a young consultant, Dr Supa, the head of the management of the Special Care Baby Unit. The hospital still retains me as a visiting professor and consultant. The Most Excellent Amina was the warrior. She represented the golden heart to push back and neutralise the reasons why the Nigerian neonates died. Like Queen Amina, the historic warrior, she distinguished herself above all her fellow First Ladies. She would be remembered wherever the story of my daunting neonatal adventures in Africa was told. She remained the heroine of the Nigerian neonates. Indeed, she was the icing on the cake of my neonatal adventure in Nigeria.

I returned to the UK and three months after my account was frozen whilst I was still in Nigeria concluding the work, I discovered that NatWest Bank had sent an apology letter regretting the ordeal they had put me through. They had unfrozen my account, but they never provided any reason why they had been so silly.

CHAPTER 16

TRIUMPH AT HADEJA

✦✦✦✦✦✦✦

The Neonatal Hospital at Hadeja had been opened and running for nearly two months. Suddenly a set of high-profile clinical visitors arrived there. This was the 'Mother and Child Health' American team of the Bill and Melinda Gates Foundation, led by a consultant neonatologist. Unknown to me, this group paid a visit to Nigeria, heard about the new Hadeja Centre and decided to visit. I was on my way to Geneva to deliver a lecture at the World Health Organisation medical devices conference 2017. I was at the West Ham London railway station waiting for a train to connect to City Airport when I received a text from The Most Excellent Amina: 'Good evening Prof. I trust you are well. We had some visitors today from the Bill and Melinda Gates Foundation who inspected our facilities, including the neonatal unit. The team leader is a neonatologist and he was so excited with what he saw that he stayed to teach resuscitation to the staff! His comment to me was that he had not seen a unit like this in Africa!! So you see prof, your dream has started to become a reality. I thought you would like to know this. Have a good night'. This message was so exciting to me.

Indeed, the Hadeja centre was not just the best in Nigeria but perhaps an exceptional one for the whole continent of Africa. The text message made my day and put me in an excellent mood as I headed off to Geneva to talk about the Hadeja Centre and my other projects at the world congress.

Many Nigerian colleagues and paediatric fellows were glad to hear the great news about the Hadeja SCBU. Reliable SCBUs in Nigeria were only available at Federal Government-owned tertiary hospitals. The majority of consultant paediatricians in Nigeria were staff of these hospitals, and were often frustrated by operating poorly-equipped SCBUs. Many of these doctors were surprised to hear that a state-owned SCBU which was not even a sub-unit of a tertiary hospital was being assessed as the best or among the best in Africa – a position no better-funded Nigerian federal teaching hospital could compete for.

The news prompted some clinicians to visit the centre to see for themselves. Dr Amina was praised at many forums for her kind gesture in spearheading such a move for the Nigerian neonate. It was noteworthy that there had been many occasions when paediatrics or nursing professionals had occupied appropriate government and political offices and positions; however, none of these had been bothered by the neonatal situation, let alone finding notable solutions as Dr Amina had done. The Hadeja centre was like no other anywhere in Nigeria, and this was widely acknowledged. The Paediatrics Forum of Nigeria (PFN) appreciated this noble gesture and decorated Dr Amina with a national honour during one of their annual conferences in recognition of her contributions to neonatal health in Nigeria.

Many not-so-happy colleagues, who felt uncomfortable that someone had crossed a professional boundary to be so highly honoured, castigated the Hadeja centre. One senior paediatrician walked up to me and said: 'Hmm Professor, I can see that this Hadeja work is quite impressive, however, I am waiting to see if it will continue to be as great after two years of service. I don't want to join in the excitement yet. You know, nothing is sustainable in this country'.

I quickly responded: 'Okay, let's wait and see, but what stops you from being happy for the neonates whilst the durability of the centre is assessed?'

The sustained standard of the neonatal centre after nearly three years of services also led to another decoration of Dr Amina by the Nigeria Association of Neonatal Care (NIANEC) during one of their national conferences.

It baffled me that people falsely believed that such an elegant and sustainable SCBU could not exist in Nigeria. If they did, why couldn't any paediatrician or any Chief Medical Director demonstrate this by pushing boundaries of limitations to create a centre of similar status in all the years before and after I joined the campaign for the reduction of Nigeria's high neonatal mortality rate? I refused to accept any excuses why organisations like the WHO, UNICEF or World Bank, in all their numerous visits, partnering and assessing progress of projects in Nigeria, never insisted on these federal government facilities showcasing a centre of such a high standard as the Hadeja centre. Perhaps it never bothered these foreign partners and their Nigerian counterparts, who were only busy going about the things that put more money in their individual pockets. One would have thought that these in-country Nigerian staff of the global organisations would not be interested in sharing the glories of the Hadeja SCBU, but this was wrong. The Hadeja centre was not typical of a Nigerian SCBU. It stood out as extraordinary. It would be an injustice against the millions of neglected Nigerian neonates for the Hadeja centre to be used as representative of a typical Nigerian SCBU. It would be a disservice and an insult to the Nigerian neonate, especially those that died, for any in-country staff of the WHO or UNICEF to showcase the Hadeja centre to their foreign partners as being a typical SCBU in Nigeria. One would not imagine this, but it happened.

The foreign partners from four different Western countries were busy taking photographs, praising the centre and its quality as they spoke to the staff: 'Nigeria has really progressed well. What you have in your centre is quite similar to what we use in our own various countries. We are impressed that Nigeria is doing very well'. What a load of nonsense! This boasting from in-country staff of the global organisation was unfounded as they were never part of the conception, design, equipping, training or setting-up of this frugal centre. How had they suddenly come to show off the very facility they knew nothing about, meeting the standard of care which they had denied the Nigeria neonates for so many years of the organisation's presence in Nigeria? Why had they chosen to deceive their international partners, using the Hadeja centre as a typical SCBU in Nigeria?

Neonatal respiratory support

I was very much aware that Nigerian special care baby units were ridden with high incidences of various dimensions of neonatal respiratory distress. I had concentrated on thermoneutrality and associated technologies for many years, carrying out scientific investigation and generating ideas to provide decisive solutions. Extreme poverty had prevented Nigerian centres from acquiring respiratory support devices in sufficient quantity to match the ever-rising need. The world had begun to celebrate my successes and the achievements of numerous neonatal thermoneutral devices and procedures. Any Nigerian centre could sustainably own a fleet of 20 or more functional incubators by applying my RIT devices and FAC programmes.

Dr Richman was a young consultant who had a personal interest in neonatal respiratory support. He had carried out a lot of studies in this area as a young consultant, but was getting more and more frustrated as he tried to find cheaper alternative technologies to ensure that neonatal mortality owing to lack of adequate respiratory support was minimised or eliminated in Nigeria.

Dr Richman approached me and recalled: 'In the past, distressed neonates were given oxygen supplements by catheterisation. We simply passed tubes through their noses and delivered pure oxygen from oxygen bottles. Few were saved, many died. We had no mechanical ventilators and any advanced systems to help. Going by what we know today, it is improper to deny these babies what the technology of this age has to offer. Neonatal mechanical ventilators cost as much as ₦15 million (about US$40,000) and it is extremely rare to find them working anywhere in Nigeria due to the high cost. We know about an alternative, a bubble continuous positive airway pressure (bCPAP) machine. This is cheaper at ₦4 million (about US$10,500) but is still unaffordable. Bubble CPAPs are in massive short supply as many hospitals have resorted to an improvised disposable version of this system. Everywhere in Nigeria, the improvised version is being used as though it is the real solution we need. The danger is that many Nigerian children today are being diagnosed with retinopathy of prematurity (RoP) as a result of the use of this deadly improvised device. This has to end somehow. Sir, I wish to request that you join us and look into this area as you have done for incubator care in this country, please.'

Dr Richman spoke with a real burden in his heart. There were other occasions when other Nigerian professionals weighed in to encourage me to consider any help possible in this area. I sympathised with them in this frustration but was not sure if this was what I wanted to delve into at the time. I was rather attracted to doing all I could to consolidate all gained achievements in neonatal thermoneutral care in the country. I was never confronted directly with this urgent need for neonatal respiratory support until a few years later.

The opportunity called for me to create a masterly display of professional artistry in setting up what would be my ideal neonatal centre for a resource-constrained setting in the city of Hadeja, Kainji state of Nigeria. The centre was proposed to have all essential devices for a modern neonatal care centre, and be fit for a high standard of practice. It would be a centre with the best assemblage of appropriate and frugal devices that could enable 'state-of-the-art' neonatal care, far above what is conventionally obtainable at a typical SCBU in Nigeria.

I was to personally source and set up the unit and its equipment. Of course I would not tolerate the use of badly-assessed devices in the range of the so-called 'improvised bCPAP'. I had to source a properly designed commercial brand of the device for use in my ideal SCBU.

I got in touch with Dr Richman for his recommendations and was surprised to hear from the doctor that he could comfortably recommend only one brand of the device, the Paykam bubble CPAP machine. He provided contact details for the sole agent of the device in Nigeria, Mr Pompay from India, and I contacted him. Mr Pompay readily gave the needed information without hesitation: 'Sir, the cost of the device in Nigeria at the present is 5.5 million naira. I have some in stock and can easily deliver to you in Hadeja whenever you are ready to pay for them.' Mr Pompay would not agree to any discount. I planned to buy only two units of the device, as it was unimaginably expensive. I was not pleased to spend a whopping ₦11 million out of the meagre funding that was available to set up the entire Hadeja SCBU, spending this on just one model of device alone.

It would take another two months after negotiations with Mr Pompay before I received the funding to place the order. I was, however, not prepared for the surprise that awaited me. Mr Pompay said over the phone: 'I am sorry to notify you, professor, that the cost of the device has gone up from the cost I originally told you. We now sell the item for 6.5 million naira. The change in price became necessary due to the poor exchange rate of the naira in recent weeks.'

'This is ridiculous, Mr Pompay!' I exclaimed: 'How could you do that? In the space of two months, you have moved the cost of such a life-saving device by 1 million naira. Do you really care about the survival of Nigeria neonates?'

'Professor, I can afford to still do this for a total of eleven million naira for the two units, just to avoid causing you an upset, but we really do sell the item for a unit cost of six and half million naira at the moment. I hope this is helpful for you,' said Mr Pompay.

'Well it is, but it's not just about me feeling upset. Nigeria neonates are dying. This system is essential, and up to 10 units are needed at each centre. At this cost no centre in this country can even afford a single unit. Is this not the reason the so-called improvised CPAP is everywhere killing neonates? Could you not renegotiate with the manufacturers of this device on behalf of these dying neonates?'

Shortly after this encounter, I travelled to Myanmar on an official scientific engagement on behalf of the Royal College of Paediatrics and Child Health. I was detailed to investigate the application of neonatal technologies for lowering neonatal mortality in this Southeast Asian country. This assignment offered me the opportunity to observe the resilience of the Southeast Asians in medical technology application. I also took notice of the great efficiency of a low-cost bubble CPAP machine in use there, a MTTS-Asia made system called the Dolphin. Upon my return to England, I did not hesitate to contact MTTS and discuss the possibilities of acquiring the Dolphin for use at the Hadeja SCBU. Hence, the Dolphin was shipped in at a discounted unit cost of 2½ million naira. This saved over 4 million naira for me to apply to acquire other systems at the new Hadeja SCBU. I later negotiated with MTTS-Asia to create avenues for making the Dolphin available to other Nigerian hospitals that might wish to procure it.

The Dolphin had many advantages over the Paykam bCPAP. Dr Richman assessed the device and was pleased to recommend its use. The news of availability of the Dolphin in Nigeria began to get round, with a few other hospitals ordering it, though in smaller quantities than were needed for the teeming numbers of distressed neonates at Nigerian centres. It was possible to have up to 10 neonates at the same time needing some kind of respiratory support in a typical Nigerian SCBU, so buying only two units of the Dolphin, even at exorbitant and unaffordable cost, could not solve the problem. The improvised CPAP was still in popular use even in places where one or two units of the Dolphin could be found. I was determined to encourage Nigerian centres to acquire the Dolphin, since this was the cheaper alternative to offer any effective support for the neonates.

It was February 2017, Dr Jumbo, the Chairman of the Neonatal Association of Nigeria (NAN), heard about the Dolphin and wanted his colleagues to know about the device. He called me and discussed his organisation's strong desire to have my presence during their forthcoming annual scientific conference in June 2017, although my very busy lifestyle could make it hard to fit the conference date into my itinerary.

'This is a very crucial meeting for us within our national practice because we hope to use the meeting to reassess the present respiratory support we are able to provide our neonates,' said Dr Jumbo. 'I believe your presence will be highly appreciated by many of our colleagues. We have also talked among ourselves at the leadership level of NAN, and we think that putting up an exhibition stand for the Dolphin will be greatly appreciated. With this, many of our attending members would be able to see the devices and assess these themselves.'

I was delighted with the idea of an exhibition stand for the Dolphin, so I hesitated no longer in accepting the invitation to attend the conference.

The conference was held in the ancient city of Kano and was well attended by participants from all over Nigeria. I flew in from England and keenly listened to as many presentations on respiratory support as possible. The more I listened the more I concluded that Nigeria neonates were still poorly supported, and hence in dire need. So many studies from different parts of the country confirmed that large numbers of Nigerian children currently suffered from retinopathy of prematurity (RoP), with a serious threat of blindness. Everyone blamed the increasing incidence of RoP on oxygen intoxication, perhaps due to the application of the improvised CPAP device in Nigeria. One presenter said: 'Our situation and the poor assistance we give to our neonates could be likened to an adult who wants to feed a child to save him from immediate hunger but ends up giving him poisoned food that kills him slowly instead'.

It was a touching conference for me. Many paediatricians really liked the Dolphin bCPAP machine but still complained that the system was too expensive for a typical Nigerian centre.

I tried to find out the ideal cost for such an important system that could encourage Nigerian practitioners to get enough units in the SCBU to completely stop the use of improvised CPAP. Most of those interviewed expected the systems to be sold for less than 1 million naira.

I felt a tap at my shoulder and turned around. It was my old friend Professor Gbenga. 'Hello Hippolite. I have been looking around for you for a chat on the respiratory devices displayed by your team,' he said.

'Hello my friend,' I replied. 'We really have got a long way to go in this issue of RoP and respiratory support devices. The few practitioners I have been able to interview on this issue have made me think that Nigerians cannot even afford the customs duties and shipping costs of this system.'

During the closing session of the conference, I sat in the front row next to Professor Gbenga. The National Chairman of NAN began to deliver his closing speech, decrying what he referred to as a very dark period in their professional history. 'This is a period when we seem to know the ugly consequences of our practice technique,' he said. 'We treat the neonate with what we can afford, but this seems to put the Nigerian child in danger of blindness. It has become clear that we do not seem to have any affordable solution to tackle the need for neonatal respiratory support. Something must be done urgently'.

The Chairman suddenly stopped speaking, looked up and removed his reading glasses. There was absolute silence in the auditorium. All eyes were fixed on him. All of a sudden, he turned his head in my direction and stared at me, and said: 'Ladies and gentlemen, what shall we do to help our neonates? We have no affordable solution or promise of any yet, even from this conference that is about to end. Professor Hippolite, what can you do for us? What can you do for Nigeria yet again?'

Wow! That was putting me on the spot. Professor Gbenga turned and looked me in the eye and laughed in reaction to the Chairman calling my name: 'Old boy, provide an answer', he said. I was rather feeling amused. Then the Chairman said: 'Seriously Professor Hippolite, I am waiting'.

'Do you really expect an answer from me?' I asked in a raised voice.

'Absolutely yes, please,' replied the Chairman, thrusting the microphone towards me.

I stood up. 'Okay then. Can you give me another half a year and I will provide an affordable solution for Nigeria,' I said and sat down. A loud ovation and clapping spontaneously erupted in the hall.

'Thank you, Professor, I am happy and we shall all look forward to this,' concluded the Chairman.

I carried out some consultations within Nigeria for a more in-depth understanding of the situation. This enabled me to begin to put my ideas together as I developed a concept for the possible bCPAP machine that could be effective and at the same time affordable to Nigerians. The idea of the Politeheart bubble CPAP machine was born. I completed my design, produced the prototype and initiated clinical trials within the promised six months. The Politeheart bCPAP was finally certified, patented and mass produced for use in Nigeria. It was a hard and gruelling task for me. Working day and night, I overstretched myself and my team to ensure that a solution was found for the neonates with as little delay as possible.

There was massive support from members of Hornchurch Baptist Church England as I updated them in my drive to continue to be relevant for these poor African neonates. They encouraged me by every means possible to bring the vision to fruition. The church dedicated one Sunday service to the display of the completed laboratory-size prototype of the device before this was sent off to Nigeria for the manufacture of the life-size prototype for clinical trials.

The success of the Politeheart was overwhelming to everyone, including me. This was the quickest product-development project I had ever completed. My non-clinical partners and I looked forward to a quick response from Nigerian hospitals and neonatologists. We expected demands and order placement to overwhelm my small group of technical staff. Everyone thought it would be hard to match production capacity to demand.

One of the first consultants to apply the Politeheart CPAP was Dr Richman. He could not hide his excitement and commented: 'Here comes the best solution so far. The system incorporates all the desired capabilities – oxygen blending, warming inspiratory channel, controllable volume flow, integrated pulse oximeter, etc, yet it can be obtained at less than 16% of the cost of Paykam CPAP system. There is no more reason for any Nigerian centre to continue to use the deadly improvised CPAP'.

This could have been true in an ideal Nigeria where the healthcare managers would become proper custodians of neonatal health. One would expect the hospital managers to go all out to make the Politeheart bCPAP available to their babies, but they never bothered. Even today, the deadly improvised

CPAP remains widely in use in Nigerian SCBUs. Only a very few hospitals are applying properly designed, commercially branded bubble CPAP. I had always argued that these hospital managers were not interested in saving the neonates – they used the high cost of the Paykam bCPAP to provide excuses for not defending the dying neonates and those they were slowly killing owing to the use of improvised CPAP. If this was not so, then one wonders why they failed to provide the neonates with proper life-saving devices when I almost single-handedly produced a device that helped to plunge the cost of the application from 6.5 million naira to as little as 0.7 million. Their priorities were rather their private pockets. The hospital managers remained one of the most powerful reasons why the Nigerian neonates died. They held the hospital purses; they were the most powerful staff; they had executive powers to do and undo; they could choose to prioritise the neonatal needs or ignore them. It is understood that the civil service 'caterpillars' at the Ministry of Health premeditated and devised wicked schemes for underfunding the hospitals; however, the hospital chief executives were responsible for the poor prioritising of the funding they had and the denial of the neonates of their rights to live! Hard talk – but this author needed to be convinced otherwise.

Corruption, conspiracies and shutdowns

In 2015, it became imperative that after my two decades of neonatal adventure I would have to transform the nature of my services, essentially requiring the discontinuation of my consultancy agreements with the hospitals. 'Empires rise and fall' is a common saying in history. How I wished this did not have to apply in the case of my bedevilled adventures for the Nigerian neonate.

At the beginning, there was much grumpy local opposition to the great job I was doing at the SCBUs. The happy winners, however, seemed to be the neonates, and in fact, the CMDs of the hospitals. The CMDs took pride in the accolades they received for nurturing functional SCBUs with growing capacities at minimal costs from abandoned materials. My consultancy drastically reduced the troubles of malfunctioning incubators, which was a huge relief to the CMDs. Those who had experienced the era of troublesome SCBU would rather suspend a disgruntled local hospital staff member than end my consultancy. Hence, efficient neonatal services still went on despite the conspiracies of destructive 'caterpillars' from works and maintenance departments, accounts and audits departments, procurement departments and administrative departments. Many immoral civil servants from these departments were used to feeding well on the so-called contractors as they inflated contracts and shared the proceeds amongst themselves. They cared little whether or not there were good patient outcomes for the money spent; what mattered most to them was their shares of the booty, to the detriment of the huge numbers of patients who died.

The lack of interest from higher government quarters in confronting and ending this wickedness was rendering the Nigerian healthcare system totally ineffective. Well-trained doctors and nurses were compelled to practise with outdated or substandard systems corruptly supplied or maintained to enrich the 'caterpillars'. Many poor patients died. The majority of enlightened Nigerians lost hope in the local hospitals and their doctors, and wished they had never gone to them for help. High death rates were blamed on 'unintelligent Nigerian doctors' rather than the caterpillars hiding in these government offices and departments. A Nigerian who could afford overseas treatment would rather go to India for treatment than allow a Nigerian doctor to operate.

I understood all this decay in the health sector and resolved to fight it in my own practice. As far as I was concerned, the integrity of my neonatal services must be protected at all costs. I resolved to leave any hospital or institution rather than allow the caterpillars to destroy the neonates under my watch. Any of my rescued SCBUs could be forced to sink by the caterpillars, but I promised myself I would leave the boat early enough, as soon as the signs appeared, rather than sink with it.

The unique successes of my consultancy were not in doubt to the caterpillars. Nevertheless, they would not accept my refusal to sanction their dishonest practices. Many resorted to blackmail, but the CMDs did not want to see a return to the ugly old days before my intervention, so their resistance would suppress the selfish agitations of the caterpillars against me. This would not last forever, as the caterpillars would retreat to plan their killing offensives, which could be launched as soon as the incumbent CMD handed over to a new, perhaps naïve successor, who might not bother to heed warnings or appreciate the poor conditions of the SCBU practice before I stepped in to turn things around. There would be a unification of efforts from the caterpillars at the SCBU, paediatrics, works, accounts and administrative departments. They all had one thing in common – unspoken grudges for lack of gratification from me, period. The unsuspecting new CMD would sink under their combined pressure, often neglecting any advice from his/her predecessor about SCBU apathy towards me.

Then the CMD would make the mistake of making an arrogant attack on my work. I would politely defend every allegation, but sternly warn against the consequences of my departure or the withdrawal of my consultancy. I would say: 'People should not be fooled into thinking that I come here for the purposes of making money. Therefore, do not attempt to harass me by threatening the legitimacy of my consultancy. I may surprise you by resigning even before you think of shutting down my consultancy. I won't be the loser; the neonates will be the losers because they will pay with their lives, sadly. How ridiculous to think that a professor from the best university in the world would come here to share in your filthy financial malpractice to the detriment of the innocent lives of neonates. I am British and a professor at a top British university; I am a decent man and if my income was not enough for me, Nigeria would certainly not be among the countries I would consider turning to.'

I knew the best time to serve my ever-ready resignation letter to any ailing CMD. I could tell from the reluctant attitude of a CMD and the frustrations that came with deliberate delay of payment of my services to the hospital. They would forget the old gloomy days of the SCBU when I had rescued them; they would forget the praises of improved outcomes from the SCBU; they would forget my risks for the hospital, which they had once praised. Selfishness and corruption suddenly blindfolded them into opting for the preventable neonatal deaths that would follow my departure. At the height of the provocation, I would resign, and the SCBU would gradually slide back into high neonatal mortality. This could take up to three years to happen at some SCBUs but less than a year in others. The nurses and doctors who worked at the SCBUs were often the first to cry out. Many of them, if they had kept my phone number, would call reporting the ugly situation and pleading for my return. Out of shame or arrogance, the patriarch CMD and his befriending caterpillars, whose failures had become evident, would find it hard to apologise or to get me back. The few CMDs whose SCBU-ensuing crises became embarrassments and threats to their jobs resorted to 'forced humility' and moves to reconcile with me, not for the sake of the neonates but to save their jobs, as in the case of Dr Brown of Eket tertiary hospital.

Extremely dishonest CMDs who were unable to unleash their wickedness against me during the prime time of their tenures smartly waited for the right time to do so. Notable among these was Dr Pumanu, the CMD of Upper Lafia Federal Hospital (ULFH). Full of evil passion, this CMD only sought to use my work for his selfish ambitions. He would not promptly pay for services rendered, and hence he feared that I would refuse to honour his request at his most needy period owing to his previous bad behaviour. He was seeking a two-year extension of his services but had to find legitimate reasons to convince his fellow immoral FMoH civil servants whose duty it was to recommend the extension.

He sat chatting with three of these fellows from the FMoH at a hotel lobby in December 2017 during a conference I also attended. 'Hello prof, come and join us briefly, please', he said to me smiling. I sat down. 'Have any of you previously met

Professor Hippolite, the globally acclaimed neonatal guru?' Showing off to the FMoH staff, he continued: 'Prof Hippolite was the expert I mentioned earlier who transformed my SCBU into the iconic unit that has become my legacy at ULFH'. This was followed by a round of handshakes from the FMoH staff in appreciation and my honour. Dr Pumanu acted in pretence, requesting an overhaul and servicing of the entire SCBU, which he had neglected for nearly two years. Aware of his previous sins, he later came to promise that he would promptly pay for the services. I was glad that I could once again be of assistance to the neonates at ULFH, so this job was executed at the agreed cost. However, in his immoral mind, he premeditated his offensive against me for refusing all his previous signals requesting a bribe. Convinced of the usual quality of my work, such CMDs knew that there might not be noticeable or obvious SCBU decays for the next two years, and they would have handed over before any major crisis developed. Therefore Dr Pumanu or a CMD like him would deliberately refuse to pay the cost of my services, hoping to compel me to come and discuss a 'cut' for them. Shamefully, they would drag this on until they handed over to a new CMD and the neonatal ordeal resumed. Dr Pumanu was a disgrace to the neonatal mission. The ULFH still has not paid for this service as I write. He was only one of a number of 'caterpillar CMDs' who conducted this evil practice against me and the neonates.

These ugly manoeuvres of that generation of CMDs and subsequent shutdowns of my consultancies made things worse for the teeming numbers of Nigeria neonates. The impact was clearly visible from a 12-year spectrum of neonatal mortality extracted from demographic publications of the WHO, NPC and the FMoH (Appendix 4). Commenting on the bar chart to an incumbent chairman of the CMDs' club, I wrote:

'Sir, factual or a coincidence but believe it or not, the trend of the sad bar chart has followed the 'highs and lows' of the aggressiveness of the national coverage of my services and collaborations with your club. My total withdrawal from your member hospitals in the last three years seems to have dragged daily mortality to a situation worse than what it was over ten years ago when the serving CMDs of your club, under the chairmanship of Professor Kature, entered into formal collaboration with me. Some aggressive intervention is urgently needed for the neonates, to push back the boundaries of neonatal deaths such as revealed by periods of Kature's and Peter's chairmanships when they consciously motivated their colleagues to invigorate our collaboration.

'I have led a team that restored confidence at a few privileged Nigerian centres. However, over 98% of local centres remain unreached; hence volumes of needy neonates continue to die. I did not achieve this by mediocrity or the so-called 'top-of-the-range' technologies from America, UK, Europe or your current new time-bomb colonial-tech master China. I did it by thinking Africa, looking around the immediate environment, researching what I could find in the local market to make functional and effective technology. This has attracted huge respect the world over. I have crossed the boundaries of engineering to earn the Fellowship of the Royal Society of Medicine of the United Kingdom (FRSM) – a no mean recognition; appointed the UK TropicalHealthEducationTrust (THET) Lecturer for 2017; the Neonatology/Perinatology Honourable Guest on the Dais

2018 in Frankfurt – first African ever to be so appointed – many times given keynote speeches on the global stage, I can go on and on, all to expose the suffering of the neonates in this country and my small frustrating efforts to drive a change. As the world celebrates and applauds such iconic inputs of medical technology in Nigeria, what do Nigerians themselves know about it? Nothing. They aren't interested. Why must Nigeria be interested, when they can always import even pencils from China and go to India to treat malaria? What a shame of a country! You copy everything other productive and proactive professors from other countries have achieved with your eyes so closed that you failed to realise that you must factor in your own peculiar dynamics such as culture, environment, climate and social disposition in your version of technology before this can become sustainable. Nigerians have refused to THINK, hence continued to SINK – pity.'

Tunde - the last man standing

The year 2014, and following, another generation of CMDs arose in Nigeria. This crop of chief executives was completely different from the era of Professor Kature and Professor Peter's CMD club committees. The FMoH caterpillars perfected another awful strategy, and their schemes brought about a generation of CMDs who cared even less for the babies. The caterpillars yet again set the dangerous scene that put the neonates in further jeopardy and neglect, exacerbating the high SCBU-based neonatal mortality rates. They were responsible for interviewing and recommending new appointees into the important office of CMD. They relegated excellence, achievements and relative qualifications of candidates to the background and instead pursued tribalism, nepotism, favouritism, bribery and corruption, which mattered more to them than the physical health of the Nigerian populace. In their insatiable craving for bribes, they demanded the deep pockets of candidates that showed interest in being nominated for appointment into the vacant posts of chief executives of tertiary hospitals. People who had paltry abilities for what the office required but who had deep pockets to pay bribes got the appointments. Better-qualified candidates who had no 'godfathers,' no money for bribes, and those who had the integrity to refuse the 'body language' signals for bribes were rejected. The result was an 'executive cowboy' era.

I regretted watching these ruthless fellows create a neonatal environment that could not sustain the SCBU successes of their predecessors. They were quick to stop the little funding that I had managed to win for the huge neonatal achievements of their predecessors. They had all the excuses in the world to legitimise their failures to uphold the SCBU standards they had inherited – 'lack of sufficient funds' was top of the list. I often wondered why they blamed this. How had their predecessors, who had inherited poor SCBUs or none at all, succeeded in building and maintaining the units' capacities they had passed on?

I believed that the primary reason these CMDs failed was lack of interest in whatever I was championing, since there was no personal financial gratification or glory from them. Whenever the opportunity arose, I would advise the CMD that the successes they could achieve in the SCBU had more to do with their personal desire and seriousness to save the neonates than the so-called government subventions. I advised them that money should be seen as a tool that could be frugally managed to save the important lives of the neonates. 'If you put money ahead of your passion for the survival of the neonates, you fail. But put passion ahead of money, and you succeed,' I would often say. However, no amount of persuasion would cause the 'lion' to let go of the 'lamb' in his teeth, and they watched shamelessly as the practice standards of their various SCBUs fell.

I could not stand watching the centres revert to increasing neonatal mortality because a CMD refused to appreciate the need to keep the SCBUs as functional as they had been when inherited. Whenever the insulting arrogance of any of the executives reached an unbearable level, I would do one of two things – I would tender my resignation to the hospital's management or suspend my consultancy to that particular hospital indefinitely. One after another, I shut down or suspended my consultancies in all the Nigerian tertiary hospitals until only one hospital was left, and only one CMD could happily say that Professor Hippolite was still an active visiting consultant or visiting professor at his hospital. This was Dr Tunde.

I began to plan 'to move on' with my African charity in new ways. I would no longer be instantly available to CMDs or crippled by legally-binding 'consultancy agreements' whose clauses the reckless cowboy CMDs never bothered to respect. Strictly speaking, I had nothing more to prove to Nigerians. I had demonstrated that SCBU success, and hence drastic neonatal mortality reduction, could be achieved using appropriately-designed home-grown technologies. I had published all my findings and they had been praised the world over. My internationally peer-reviewed techniques had enriched the global scientific and global health communities. I had used the past 22 years of my practice to personally demonstrate my sciences and research to Africans. The decision to apply these for self-sustenance was for Africans to make.

My efforts to train more Nigerian technicians along the lines of my practice were not as successful as the clinical outcomes. The technicians looked away from the technologies because they could not see immediate personal financial enrichment from them – the get-rich-overnight syndrome; hence, the years of learning whilst I was around were wasted. Therefore the technicians at each local hospital could not provide effective help when I withdrew. Hence, only a few years from the withdrawal date, neglect by careless CMDs would start to result in visible disasters at the SCBUs. Some CMDs with this emerging need would wish to revert to me for help. Unfortunately, they were too late. I had moved on. The redefinition of my African work required all remaining legal entrapments in the name of 'consultancy agreements' to be dismantled. The sun was setting on the once happy collaborative successes of the CMDs' club with me. The cries of the neonates echoed across the approaching darkness with no one to rescue them.

'Worrying times are ahead,' responded the only man standing, Tunde. It was the cry of a man who was truly compassionate for the continued survival of the Nigerian neonates.

'Quite frankly Prof,' Tunde said, 'I do not wish to selfishly impede your future if I must plead with you to change your mind, but we will miss you greatly at our SCBU. Your legacy in neonatal healthcare in Nigeria cannot be easily equalled or forgotten'. Tunde's SCBU was, in fact, about the smallest in capacity in the country. His predecessor in office, Dr Elesh, had decided to liaise with me to make this one of the most functional SCBUs in Nigeria irrespective of its size, and he had succeeded. Just like many of his colleagues at the present CMD club, Tunde watched as his predecessor and I literally transformed their formerly shoddy SCBU into a centre they could be proud of, and which the hospital management was always willing to showcase to visitors, irrespective of its size. What was fascinating about Tunde was exactly what I had expected his CMD Club colleagues – successors to the previous generation of CMDs – to do. It was Tunde's resolve to do everything managerially possible to improve on the standard of the SCBU he had inherited, the least of which would be to maintain the inherited standard even in the unlikely worst situation of poorer funding.

Tunde matched action to desire and often held meetings with me, jointly brainstorming on the best methods that could reduce cost without reducing the unit's standards. Tunde was properly rewarded because at the time when his other colleagues were losing professional accreditation of their centres for postgraduate training in paediatrics due to dwindling SCBU standards, his own SCBU enabled his hospital to achieve full accreditation by all relevant professional bodies for the very first time in the history of his hospital. Tunde did not achieve this because he had better funding than the rest of the hospitals; in fact, his funding was one of the poorest in the country. His success was as a result of his humility, interest and passion to ensure that the unit remained functional enough for the neonates to survive. The success had little to do with money or availability of government funding subventions. I was proud of Tunde's achievement and congratulated him.

After 22 years of bold, consistent and unparalleled intervention in the creation of effective solutions for neonatal survival, I made an announcement. This was orchestrated by an unpleasant chain of events necessitating a change. I reacted to the occasion by sending out a letter to the last man standing, Dr Tunde:

'I am now writing you in three capacities – as a personal friend, and as the CMD of a hospital where I am presently offering neonatal consultancy services or where I hold a visiting consultant position. I also write to you because you are a top Nigerian manager with a passion for the survival of Nigerian neonates. There are only three of you I so consider and hence I independently write for your active advice and intervention.

'The CMDs' club has, no doubt, been a great partner in my revolutionary intervention in Nigeria's neonatal healthcare for over 20 years. I am thankful to God for the actions of Prof Kature and his CMDs' club executives in formalising this collaboration many years ago, and also gazetting this in one of your white papers from your Benin City conference of that year. As the whole world of global health continues to celebrate the successes of my bold unconventional adventure which has impacted every regional and cultural part of Nigeria, the CMDs' club and all members who allowed their neonates to have access to the technologies must position themselves to take accolades for so doing. Nothing lasts forever, and that includes practice in this capacity. It has been 22 years since I

took up this challenge, starting from Mbong Teaching Hospital in 1996. I also feel this is the right time to wind up my current style of assistance in Nigeria. I will be calling on each of the three of you for private discussions to explain the details of my present situation which has necessitated this move. I will also be happy to provide a smoother way for your individual hospitals to cope with the immediate changes that my withdrawal might bring. Recent events at my primary base – the Royal University London, where I hold a professorial position – as well as the current state of corporate Nigeria have a lot to do with this move. Please bear with me and expect my call this weekend for further updates on this issue.'

I was also pleased to send notifications to many of the global health organisations that had honoured my contributions. One of these was a letter to Elana and Adronusa:

'I am delighted to write to appreciate the roles you have played in keeping me in the Global health network of the World Survival Organisation (WSO) ever since your 'radar' captured my ambitious Nigerian work amongst the neonates. It has been almost 22 years since this work began. I am happy that my rising profile at Royal University London over the years did not alter my passion and drive to push the boundaries of neonatal survival in Nigeria. You are well aware of this fact. However, I sense that this is now about to change significantly. I have decided to share with you a very condensed summary of this work and the proposals for its future transformation as I have prepared this for the International Relations Office of Royal University London. Please find this attached. I would

appreciate it if you can always remember that I am available to serve on any of your committees and gatherings wherever my wealth of knowledge could be assessed to be useful. I am reasonably confident that I have a lot to deliver in the drive to end high neonatal mortality rate in low- and middle-income countries of the world through essential appropriate devices and technologies. I earnestly covet your continued friendship and any reasonable introductions. Meanwhile, I am still waiting for my place of work to come up with the way forward in order to leverage on the huge successes I generated in the last twenty years.'

I also received an invitation from my constituency's Member of Parliament, Jessy Loperma MP, when she gladly requested me to summarize my services to the Nigerian neonates. This invitation and the following meeting were uniquely timed, as I considered that it was wise to ensure that my ambassadorial services as a British citizen were well documented, even if unrewarded. Hence I did not hesitate to accept the invitation to the MP's surgery.

CHAPTER 17

THE INTERVIEW

✦✦✦✦✦✦✦

In my official capacity, I was invited by the International Partners' Office (IPO) of Royal University to be interviewed about issues relating to my Nigerian work. A condensed summary of my activities was produced and submitted to the office.

Do I have any regrets? Yes, there are many. Asked about the most regrettable incident, I said, 'If you think this has anything to do with the doctors or nurses, then you will be disappointed, because it does not. If you also think I will begin to talk about the hopelessness of the civil servants at the Nigerian Ministry of Health, then you are completely wrong. Indeed, you would think I would regret involving some disgruntled paediatricians who viewed me as a professional 'gatecrasher' coming in from nowhere and stealing all the attention. Or you might expect me to regret the grumpy maintenance engineers who feared that a self-acclaimed expert had come from nowhere to expose their inefficiency. It was difficult dealing with the often parochial views of such individuals who neither made good things happen nor allowed better people to make things happen. I was never totally surprised at their roles, even after scoring an unprecedented success in my 'unconventional' cost-effective techniques.'

'Expecting to change a grown man whose mind is set on selfish interests is like bending a spring and expecting it to remain in the same position when you let go of it. There must be a better strategy for a permanent and sustainable responsible workforce in Nigeria. This country lacks the appropriate labour capacity for the necessary change. Sad indeed.'

A long silence followed as I looked up and down the room.

'Who has to do with this greatest regret of yours?' I was asked.

'I wish the university system was better than the Ministry and the hospital administrations in Nigeria, then there would have been hope from hundreds of half-baked graduates being churned out every year by institutions of higher learning in this country. The universities are run by pseudo-politicians whose passion is money-making and everything except global academic excellence. The system is full of academically-retarded individuals brandishing worthless titles and waiting for their opportunities to fulfil their insatiable selfish interests. I have spent over a quarter of a century of my life in full-time academic studies, from primary school through to my last work as a postdoctoral student. These were the foundational years of all the achievements I recorded for the Nigerian neonate. The hospital people marvelled at the ease with which I solved their crippling SCBU problems, especially respiratory support and thermoneutral complications. They wished their own in-house engineers could be so skilful, but never bothered to think about the universities that produced them. I regret that the universities are incapable of producing quality technical personnel with a passion for the reduction of patient mortality rather than for having the fattest bank accounts. I thought I could correct this before winding up my Nigeria work, or before I lacked the strength for long hours at work. I thought I could walk into the universities and correct things from the grass roots. The vice-chancellors and university authorities I encountered were visionless, and full of mediocrity and selfishness – they were too short-sighted to figure out the depressing future of medical technology in Nigeria. They failed to understand the urgency. The vice-chancellors and their worthless institutions – they form my greatest regret.' I sat back, feeling a deep sense of disappointment.

On several occasions, I looked on in disbelief whilst university academics talked about the successes of their colleagues. They would talk about their material possessions but never about their academic outputs, like high references of high impact international journal publications, scientific discoveries and research spin-off products. These were completely lacking in the list of what constituted the successes of a Nigerian academic professor. He was instead respected and praised for the kind of house he had built, the cars he could purchase and how gorgeously and expensively he dressed, irrespective of how he had cheated the system to acquire his wealth. The wrong yardstick was used to measure academic success and what inspired the younger generation. Therefore the research institutions were completely ineffective and had no drive to grow their own technologies.

I understood that the universities held a crucial key to generating the appropriate workforce to tackle the inefficient total dependency of the Nigerian healthcare system on 'black box' foreign technologies. I had carefully observed the abilities of so many instrument technicians and engineers that tried to handle neonatal devices across the Nigerian hospitals. I concluded that most of them lacked knowledge of the fundamental theories and basic physics behind the operation of the various devices. The devices were simply 'black boxes' to so many of them. Hospital management cherished the immediate positive impacts of my presence wherever I was appointed as visiting consultant. Some hospital chiefs wanted the successes I brought but wished they did not have to pay me for my work, since I would not let them defraud the system.

The Head of the Works Department of Efeko Federal Hospital would fight back. He persuaded the deputy CMD to orchestrate a secret understudy of my skill so as to sack me as soon as the members of his 'maintenance staff' had finished learning from me. This was agreed. Therefore he appointed two of his maintenance staff and detailed them to 'always stay with the doctor to secretly learn from whatever he does that so easily makes the systems work. We can sack him afterwards and save all the money we pay to keep him here'.

The plan was finalised and I was told that two engineering staff had been posted to 'supervise' me whenever I was on duty.

This sounded strange to me but never bothered me. I had no clue that they were to be my secret students or spies. 'That's okay with me if this is what you want. I will always alert them whenever I am at work,' I replied. The two men would ask the most stupid technical questions on earth at the wrong times, and since I was not told they were my students, I would normally ignore such questions to avoid distractions. Nevertheless I provided them with answers when the questions were asked at the right times. The result was that the more they observed, the more confused they became. They were also too impatient to stay with me for the entire duration of a visit. Whenever they were alerted to come over for my session, they would arrive more than two hours after work had already started and would spend 10-30 minutes only before going away, so they never understood what was going on. They were simply not interested in calmly paying attention, let alone understanding my technical judgements.

I visited this centre every six months, spending an average of ten days per visit. This implies only 20 days per year of my physical presence. Given that these unwilling engineering staff stayed with me for no more than 30 minutes a day, they would have tried to understudy me for only a period of 10 hours in a year. How ridiculous! These fellows intended to spend ten hours studying a skill I had learnt over 15 years of post-graduation continuous schooling. Many other centres tried this technique, but they all failed.

I had made myself an excellent teacher over the years and was always ready to pass my knowledge on to other willing and passionate individuals. I always emphasised that the secret of my success was not my technical know-how but my undiluted passion to save the neonates. I was a good planner who wanted to appropriately integrate a systematic way of grooming would-be students for the transfer of my skills. Quite a number of young men joined me for this, often from the open Nigerian labour market. Only a few understood my vision and drive. Many joined me because they thought this fellow from England might have some money and could quickly make them rich. They soon got disappointed when the cash did not flow as anticipated, and left.

Some others wanted to learn but did not want complicated skills that would take a long time to acquire. Emadus was one such technical assistant who would not follow my precepts and study plan. He was in a hurry and would often abandon what he had been detailed to do to try other technical jobs he had not yet graduated into doing. In the process he endangered the lives of neonates many times, earning himself a lot of queries. Emadus made extraordinary demands for unearned money, hence exposing his real intentions for joining my team. He wanted to quickly understand all about my trade so as to float his own independent organisation for incubator repairs. I would have liked this, but I believed that Emadus's love of money would make him compromise the lives of the neonates with dishonest chief executives and in-house hospital engineers.

I quite often suggested that CMDs should officially assign a permanent in-house maintenance man to my team to undergo a well-tailored five-year training programme that was capable of ensuring the functional sustainability of their incubator systems, especially to prevent the SCBU crashing whenever I found it necessary to withdraw my services. Only a very few CMDs cared enough to heed this advice. Some others did, but the assigned technical staff and their immediate line managers were not dedicated enough to make the most of the short time when I was present. Years would roll by before the management, and even the staff in question, would realise that he had not been able to learn any substantial skills.

I felt sorry for one such in-house staff member, Mr Aliyu of Mubi Federal Hospital. Aliyu always struggled to make his line manager understand that he needed to be completely excused from other duties for the entire eight days that I would normally spend at their hospital during each of my two visits in the year. It took over three years before this could sink into the manager's consciousness. Aliyu had evidence that his manager would not let him spend enough time to undergo my training schedules.

I clearly noticed the moment when Aliyu began to show the signs of the neonatal compassion which I considered a prerequisite for effective learning, and I intensified my encouragement. It was quite clear that most of the so-called biomedical engineers at the Nigerian hospitals had never studied human anatomy or physiology, let alone understood the physics of the human-machine interface that was supposed to be fundamental to medical systems design and maintenance. I was prepared to use the emerging zeal shown by Mr Aliyu to fill in the gaps and build upon it – this would take some time, but I was used to being patient in this kind of situation. Mr Aliyu often goofed, but this never bothered me as I continued to encourage him. Many of the CMDs were not as patient as me. They wanted to see these technicians become as skilled as me and display all my technical abilities in three years – a non-graduate technician displaying the skills of a professor with many years of experience!

Poor Aliyu; his impatient CMD was quoted as referring to him as 'a dull unintelligent man, incapable of significant skills to show for the years of following the professor. He must have had a low APGA score at birth'. That was a mean and arrogant comment to make concerning someone whom I knew was working hard to step up his game after many years of frustration with his colleagues.

I finally came to terms with the realisation that putting this 'new wine' of my technical skills into the 'old bottles' of these inflexibly money-hungry old Nigerian technicians, engineers and doctors could yield little or no change. 'Going to the universities to capture the unstained young brains, to inspire them and properly train them in readiness for what they would later encounter at the hospitals could be my best sustainable solution for Africa,' I said to my mentor, Professor Harry.

'What do you mean? A kind of university collaboration?' asked Professor Harry.

'Exactly, but I am thinking of something more than a simple collaboration. I wish I could assemble all my fragmented training modules at all the teaching hospitals in a central university. I could then leverage this to design a proper human capacity-building centre that could target the creation of a new and effective breed from young university students,' I said.

'Great! This sounds brilliant to me, Hippolite. Our Department can always support this move. Let me know how this progresses and what you would like the Department to do for you to ensure the success of the move.'

My wealth of experience of the exact practical needs of the neonatal healthcare field of practice would influence the programmes, courses and modules I would set up from the foundation. Eight Nigerian universities became aware of the proposed capacity-building project and applied for the role of the local academic collaborator for this. The Bioengineering Department of Royal University finally approved the government-owned Ikenga University to host my work in Nigeria. Ikenga University thus signed a memorandum of understanding, and hence, officially entered into a collaboration agreement with Royal University. This was a milestone achievement for the vice chancellor of Ikenga University, Professor Aloyston, as many other Nigerian universities competitively applied for this collaboration.

Professor Harry and I were disappointed during the first two years of this collaboration as Nigeria's unstable character reared its head again, limiting the smooth take-off of the project. The agreement establishing the collaboration had aspects to be fulfilled by the Royal University and also those to be fulfilled by Ikenga University. I designed the rigorous steps for the screening of postgraduate candidates to be jointly supported by the two universities. These were, however, undermined by the crafty senior staff of Ikenga University who were involved in the process. Each person manipulated his way to push forward their favoured relations for interview and prevented the best candidates from being shortlisted for the interview processes. I was disappointed and deeply regretted choosing Ikenga University for this role. The university could not even fulfil their other obligations of the MoU, thereby forcing the Royal to cancel the slots reserved for these Nigerian students.

In another related opportunity, Ogbete University shamelessly supplied postgraduate candidates who could not write comprehensive 'statements of purpose', which were a mandatory step during the first stage of screening for admission into the Royal. I investigated the poor interview performances of the candidates and found that they were presented because they were the Vice-Chancellor's candidates and not because of any academic excellence.

The university's professor in charge of postgraduate studies, Prof Okuku, tried to justify the move. He asked me to explain to my Royal colleagues that these candidates were his VC's choice and, hence should be accepted for admission. I was furious at such low professional esteem of a professor, and replied: 'Do you expect the prestigious Royal University to be as shameless as your university and admit no-brainers?' The candidates were, of course, rejected and refused admission. Nigeria tried to manipulate everything and wrongly thought this was how big global institutions like the Royal University were run – wrong.

Professor Harry was giving up on Nigeria, but I was shamed big time by these clueless pseudo-politicians at the helm of the affairs of Nigerian universities. The brick walls at these universities were my frustration and deepest regret.

I turned my anger at every opportunity against the lack of professionalism, excellence and fairness in the education sector, arguing that these factors had led to academic laziness, poor industrial output and lack of creative minds in Nigeria's workforce. These factors bred professional engineers and scientists who had plenty of time to complain against the government but no time to think, design or create.

As these issues burned in my heart, I received a rare invitation to be a guest speaker at Nigeria's National Engineering Centre Abuja to address 'engineering in medical practice'. My lecture threw up mind-blowing concealed truths, threw jibes on Nigeria's folly, put engineers on the spot for corruption and laziness and challenged the sincerity of the so-called international aids to Nigeria. It was electrifying. Lots of journalists wanted to field private questions at the end of the speech.

One of these was: 'What advice do you have for the government on ways to create a conducive environment for engineers to become effective in Nigeria?'

I replied: 'I have no advice for the government, but I have some for the engineers. They are not unproductive because of the government's attitude but because they are lazy, dishonest, scientifically uncreative and have loads of excuses to justify failure rather than good ideas for success. Engineers are conversant with boundary conditions in mechanics and designs, right? They should learn from this. They should stop complaining about poor grid electricity, poor government, poor transport etc.; they should rather regard these situations as 'boundary conditions' in order to focus on the other scientifically alterable factors that could yield them some successes. There are exciting climatic, environmental and natural factors in this country that government policies cannot touch or influence; they should focus on these with their scientific zest, if they've got any, with a view to harnessing them for effective engineering solutions. Then they would create successes. Then they would become stars and be celebrated. Then their successes would inspire those failing at governance and other services. Then Nigeria would become better and better. Then you journalists would give me some break from your endless lopsided journalism in this country.'

ONE MAN, MANY TITLES

✦✦✦✦✦✦✦

I was given many titles and nicknames in the course of my neonatal career in Nigeria. Some of these were quite funny and occasioned by my character, unassuming attitude and humility. It was quite obvious that many of the negative ones were never openly used by the individuals or groups of people who invented them. It was not surprising that someone like me could be given so many names as I really pushed the boundaries of the operational norms at the hospitals, especially with the Management and Accounting Departments – I spent my time with the neonates on the wards and never gave bribes, never connived to 'pad up' maintenance bills, never agreed to alter financial figures for the benefit of dishonest staff, never went after favour-seeking whilst on duty. These were what mattered most to many senior and junior civil servants at the hospitals, but I refused to do them.

They tried to hit back at me by precipitating frustrating circumstances. They delayed the processing of my bills and payments as my files would suddenly go missing, the payback from immoral and disgruntled bribe-seeking civil servants. My bills would go for months, even years, without being processed or paid. Some of my nicknames came as a result of my resilience against these forces, and my kindness. The Yobe people of Nguru called me a name in the Hausa language that translated as 'MD's white man', due to my generosity, ingenuity, accuracy and dependability.

Some Kano hospital staff were disappointed that I refused to notice their 'body language' asking for cash gifts, so they nicknamed me the 'shrewd Igbo man'. To so many, I represented different things. Some nurses who did not know me so well described me as 'that technician that comes to repair the incubators at the SCBU'. At Benin City, they nicknamed me the 'funless man' because some people felt I had time for nothing but neonatal work. I would often not bother to react to such wrong impressions about me, to the utter amazement of the local staff who knew me a bit better than others. They would be more interested in offering to correct these impressions, but I would pretend not to notice and moved on with my business.

I was used to dressing so simply that it was not easy to distinguish me. I never wore suits and well-ironed jackets to the neonatal wards, as many local professors would. A young doctor once walked up to me at Abuja to seek a piece of advice, but had a confession to clear up first: 'Your manner of dressing does not make it easy to identify you, sir,' said the young lady.

'I don't understand what you mean,' I replied.

'I was here yesterday to meet you. I sat in the waiting area whilst you were teaching and doing your ward round inside the SCBU with your resident doctors and other students. The nurses asked me to sit beside the gowning room so I could see you when you come out to deposit your gown, assuring me that you were going to finish at 2 pm. I was sitting right beside the gowning room, expecting to see someone dressed like our local professors, but I was wrong; I saw you all right when you hung up your gown, but hesitated to come up to you as I felt this could not be the highly-acclaimed Professor Hippolite. You were dressed more like one of the resident doctors who were hanging up their gowns at the end of your rounds with them. After half an hour, the nurse came up to me to ask if I had finished with 'the professor'. She described you and I knew that I had missed the opportunity, because I had misplaced your personality. Prof, I really love how simple you are'.

In the midst of these conflicting impressions and the name-calling, I was an excellent 'doctor' to so many. During a continental conference of paediatricians in Lagos, I sat quietly beside an exhibition stand where my products were displayed. A very senior clinician came by with a small group of friends and began to ask questions about my devices to the marketing agents. He obviously did not recognise that I was the person sitting beside the booth. He had encountered me many years earlier during his days as a resident doctor at one of the teaching hospitals at Benin. He began to tell his friends about the special character of the doctor who designed the products that they were admiring.

'Have you met Professor Hippolite in person?' asked his colleague.

'Yes, he was a visiting consultant at my unit many years ago when I was a resident doctor,' he replied. The doctor talked about my perfect understanding of thermoneutral control in the neonate and my accurate predictions of outcome during practice in the ward: 'This man personally impressed and inspired us during those days whenever he walked into the ward and examined the patients we were treating. He could look at the incubator, notice something wrong, then peeped through the canopy to look at the baby and turned around to yell out: 'who is managing this baby without his active mind? This baby is thermally unstable – check it out'. And I tell you, he would always be right when we checked. That guy was an excellent doctor who inspired many us'.

To some other people I was a brilliant teacher. Doctor Chuks was a senior registrar as a resident doctor at Enugu when he enrolled in his first course of paediatrics incubation technique of which I was the resource person. Many years after graduation, Chuks recounted his experience: 'Professor Hippolite knew how to take you back to basic secondary school physics, using this to explain the complex thermoneutral conditions of a neonate. He was the person that dispelled the aura of magic I used to feel with the neonatal incubator towards the end of my residency training. I will not forget how, during my course days, we saw him tear down the incubator in a short time and put the whole thing together again as we watched, all in the attempt to show us that it was a system we could understand if we wished to. He would often say: 'hey guys you can see, you've got no witch inside this box playing the game – it's all about physics, cables and elements'.'

I was seen by many as the professor who had a very good understanding of what he professed – thermoneutral complications in the neonate. Above all these titles was the one given by a set of people that viewed me differently. I was invariably motivated by a divine calling based on my understanding of how God communicated with me. I would go into dangerous places where many other professionals were afraid to go, just because I felt God had sent me there. I would choose to remain quiet about my itinerary because I had sensed that a listener would discourage me from embarking on my intended mission. Just a mention of some intended locations in dire need of help in the country, and people quickly tried to discourage me: 'That area is dangerous, please don't go there'.

I was once carrying out my routine consultancy visit at the tertiary hospital in Yola city, Adamawa State. One morning I decided to send an email to a senior friend of mine who was serving in the United Nations as a medical staff member at Afghanistan during the Afghan war days. I wrote: 'Uncle Jones, I just remembered you this morning and wanted to know how you are doing... I am carrying out my routine tour at the Federal tertiary Hospital Yola at the moment.' I was shocked that within five munities of hitting the 'send' button, Uncle Jones wrote back: 'What? That means you are working in Adamawa. I am scared, that place is 'dangerous-o', so be careful and conclude it quickly and leave that area'. This was a guy in Afghanistan during the days of incessant bombing telling another person in a relatively peaceful country to quickly depart from a 'dangerous' place. Ironic, wasn't it?

I understood the sincere concerns of my loved ones, but I preferred to spare them their fears for my safety for the long duration of each routine tour. Therefore I kept my places of duty silent from many people, including my wife and my mother. I ensured that only my bosom friend, Ogene, was kept informed of my movements within Nigeria. Many referred to me as the 'charity worker' who risked his life for the Nigerian neonates. To the members of my Hornchurch Baptist Church Essex, who supported my 'charity' in Africa, I was simply a steadfast 'missionary'.

My PhD research was a very expensive programme that has been narrated earlier in this book. It was one of the great successes of Professor Harry's group which independently produced eleven scientific journal papers in international journals. Once during one of the Royal's scientific conference poster displays and competitions my project was among the few chosen for public view. Every chosen presenter was mandated to insert the logo or names of the organisations or individuals responsible for funding their research. My poster stood out as it was the only one with 'unknown' or unidentifiable names of sponsors. My insertion was, 'This project has been funded by 'The Father Unlimited". I was unashamed to state the obvious when assessors questioned me on this, 'Who is this and in what country is this organisation?' I was asked. I simply pointed my finger upwards and responded, 'The Father unlimited in heaven above'. This was followed by laughter from some of the panel members. 'Impressive, I knew it! Hippolite you are never short of inspiring words' said one of the assessors.

God did it all

It will be a terrifying situation for me if I do not carefully render to God all His full glory for all that transpired in my daunting adventures passing through the Royal and standing firm in my fight for the Nigerian neonate. I did not suddenly acquire the strong character and experience that enabled me to take this step for the neonates. Therefore it became necessary to narrate and put straight records on how God, the omnipotent, did what no man could do for me, and hence this success story. Some people who neglect the opportunity to help others and be proud to announce it often resort to fabrication and lies in order to 'keep up appearances'. Such lies are told so repeatedly to deceive many hearers that the peddler completely forgets that it was in the first place fabricated and untrue, especially if the lies are unchallenged.

Everyone likes to identify with success but not everyone likes to get 'dirty' and make sacrifices to produce a success. I believe it is my duty as the person at the centre of the actions to assist those who would trust God to narrate how it all happened, and who did it. This awesome God whom I serve was entirely unassisted – 'the only unseen drummer that produced the tune of the music I danced'. He remains my superhero. He defied the unwillingness of those that were capable of helping and went on to orchestrate the unsual route that produced the neonatal passion and excellent professional practice I possess.

Before the blossom

This aspect of my story has become necessary as it would

be improper to relegate God to the background of this story, especially as it relates to the fundamental events that transformed me into the neonatal service. The journey began even before I knew what it would become.

Immediately after the completion of my National Youth Service (NYSC), I returned to the city of Onitcha, where my second eldest brother, Donald, lived. Donald was much junior to our eldest and about 12 years my senior. He was fond of me and treated me as dearly as his own younger brother, so we were very close. I loved spending my holidays with him when I was still in school. Donald was a very rich businessman, who could easily have assisted my academic progress all on his own if he had wanted to do so.

I lost my biological father when I was still a toddler. I lived with my maternal grandmother and later my mother's younger sister until my year 4 primary school stage, when I returned to my mother in Ekeuku village. My elder brother, Chubuks, who was about three years younger than Brother Donald, was kind enough to take over the payment of my school fees until I finished secondary school. It was an immense sacrifice as Chubuks worked hard to bear the costs all alone. Chubuks loved me greatly and was very proud of my intelligence. Unlike Brother Donald, he was selfless, working hard to provide for the entire family. He ensured that the rest of our siblings continued with their education, being exclusively responsible till they completed their tertiary education. He toiled day and night as a trader and sacrificially denied himself a lot of youthful pleasures just to ensure he saved enough for the schooling of his siblings. He was indeed a blessing, deserving the great rewards that only God could give. Brother Chubuks, all on his own, sponsored my last three years in primary school, entire secondary education, and was prepared to go ahead with the funding of my university education. Chubuks was exceptional for me!

In his own ways, Brother Donald was a great encouragement to me, promising to send me to the university as well. I was very close to both of them. All along my father's younger brother, whom I later entitled 'Papa,' admired my developing personality and resolved to begin to contribute towards my progress in life. Without declaring his intentions, Papa invited me to spend my final secondary school holiday with his family in the city of Uyo where he lived. When I was set to return to school, Papa asked for the cost of my university entrance examinations, called 'JAMB', and handed over the full amount of money to me in addition to some pocket money.

I passed the university entrance exam and was set to begin my undergraduate training in mechanical engineering. Papa called me and delivered the good news, saying: 'It is my intention to offer a helping hand to Chubuks in funding your university education. You need to open a bank account. You should learn how to calculate your expected annual living costs, tuition and other fees to prepare your yearly budget. This should adequately cover your school fees, accommodation and feeding with a little for miscellaneous expenditure. When it's done, you should pass your budget to me first and I will always give you part of the money to put in your bank account so you can afterwards go to Chubuks for him to give you the balance'.

After the budget funding of the first year of the expected five years of my study, it was clear to me what Papa's full intention was. I had returned to the city of Uyo with my first budget to see Papa before my departure for my first year at the Enugu University. Papa collected the pieces of paper from me, read through the budget and began to advise me on how I must remain disciplined to ensure a good future for myself as an undergraduate in faraway Enugu. It was a message well-delivered with great love, and I could feel this.

Papa finally went into his bedroom with the pieces of paper. On coming out he handed over a bundle of money to me and asked me to count it. I did and it amounted to a little more than 60% of the total budget submitted to him.

'Thank you sir,' I said.

'Okay, this is how I want to be doing it for the rest of your remaining four years of undergraduate studies. You can now go to Chubuks and explain to him so he could provide you with the balance,' Papa said. Donald again did not bother to assist Chubuks in providing the balance of the support I needed.

Papa was a much-disciplined surgeon and an excellent 'father' to me. Chubuks was happy for Papa's gesture and later thanked him for his kindness.

Many years earlier when Papa was a boy, my biological father, Nnoka, had also played some supportive roles in various ways in Papa's life. It was a nice thing for Papa to have learnt the act of kindness from Nnoka, and now I must learn the same thing from Papa. Papa and Chubuks were both men of excellent heart, playing the roles my late father had left behind. With carefully-crafted and sustained budgeting, both men diligently supported my undergraduate studies.

As the years went by Papa and I were becoming ever closer to each other. Papa was paying as much attention to me as a biological father, so a stronger bond began to develop. Papa promised to send me for postgraduate studies at his former university in Heidelberg, Germany. Unfortunately, by the end of my NYSC in 1989, the Nigerian economy had become so damaged that Papa was unable to fulfil this promise due to financial constraints. However, his dreams for my progress had already inspired a desire in me to strive to go further for more academic qualifications.

I was finishing my NYSC when my former university professor and project supervisor notified me that I had been offered admission to commence my Master's Degree programme at the university. I shared the good news with Papa and Donald but was unsure if brother Donald was still interested in funding my further studies. Brother Chubuks had played such a huge fatherly role in my life as he single-handedly paid for my education up to the end of secondary school before Papa teamed up with him in funding my undergraduate education. I didn't wish to bother him any longer. Papa was obviously no longer as financially buoyant as he used to be; however, my big brother Donald's business at Onitcha was doing very well.

I chose to return to Onitcha, where Donald lived, to see what would become of my immediate plan to return to the university to commence my postgraduate work. At various times I opened up discussions with my brother concerning my pending MSc admission at Enugu, but there was no suggestion from Donald that he was interested in funding this. My former undergraduate coursemates were beginning to get jobs in the booming oil and gas industry in Nigeria, but I was unwilling to apply for a job yet, hoping that Donald would soon ask me to take up my MSc admission.

Some months passed, and the MSc dream was fading. Finally I decided to submit some applications for employment. I discussed this with Donald several times to see if I would be discouraged from taking such a step, but Donald kept saying it was okay. It was not long before I was invited by Shell Petroleum Development Company for an interview in Port Harcourt. The interview ended late in the evening, and it was too late to start a journey back to Onitcha. I had no one to spend the night with in Port Harcourt, and the city of Uyo was closer, so I decided to spend the night there with Papa.

Papa had returned from his evening rounds at the hospital, had had his dinner and was reclining in the sitting room when I walked in.

'Good evening sir,' I greeted.

Papa turned in surprise: 'Where have you come from this late, Hip?' he asked. I explained.

'Why did you change your mind about the admission that Professor Ofodile obtained for you?' asked Papa. 'Is it with such a basic degree as a BSc that you wish to start life?' He frowned.

'Not so, sir. I have been in Onitcha ever since I returned from NYSC in Baguda State. I thought brother Donald would fund me but since this has been delayed beyond the start date of the MSc programme I decided to think of starting a career, perhaps with Shell.'

Papa enquired whether the admission slot was still open for me by telephoning Professor Ofodile that night. 'Oh yes, doctor,' said the professor. 'If Hippolite is still interested, our department will be happy for one of our best undergraduate students ever to return for his MSc with us. I can make it happen. He only needs to come and pay his tuition fees and register immediately. I am sure he is capable of catching up with his mates who have already started.'

Standing up, Papa said: 'Go to the kitchen and let them give you food to eat. I will be right back'. He went upstairs to his bedroom and returned after about an hour. I had finished eating. 'Come and sit down here next to me,' he said to me. Seated, he handed over a bundle of money to me and said: 'This is the full amount of your MSc tuition fees as Professor Ofodile told me earlier. You need to go to bed now so you may leave for Enugu very early in the morning in order to arrive in good time for the registration process. Good night'.

I was full of excitement. I completed my registration before close of work the same day and headed back to Onitcha. I told my brother all that happened and how I ended up in Enugu. Donald felt challenged by Papa's kindness because he knew he was rich enough to help me. 'Okay, that is so kind of Izume. Since he has paid the tuition completely, do not go back to him for your maintenance costs, come to me instead,' Donald ordered me.

It was an 18-month MSc degree programme. I completed it and began my career as a self-employed medical engineer, developing my range of medical laboratory devices. The more I progressed in this largely unknown field of practice, the more I desired to embark on overseas further studies, perhaps for a PhD degree to enhance my competitive advantage. I hoped to get into a university in the USA, then Canada, then the United Kingdom. My brother Donald was believed to be rich enough to fund this. Some of my friends were getting married, but I would have been stupid to start a family when this ambition of travelling for further studies was still alive. It could hamper any travel.

I was still hopeful that my brother would fund me if I got the admission. Donald had some connections in Europe via his in-law and in Australia via a friend. These people used their foreign currency to assist me with exam registration costs and some books to enable me to study for GRE and other overseas exams so that I could apply for a PhD course. Donald would discuss it with these fellows and arranged how he would refund them. However, what surprised me most was that my brother would later compel me to give back the local currency equivalent of the costs to him in spite of making the foreign fellows believe he would be the person to fund the course. There was no such expenditure that Donald did not recover from me, so this generated a lot of doubt whether Donald would really support me even if I got the admission.

I used every opportunity to test if I was wasting my time waiting to travel for this PhD. I got green lights of admission from institutions like the University of Ontario, Canada and Massachusetts Institute of Technology USA, but had to look away from these pursuits because it was clear that neither Papa nor Donald had the funds or was willing to pay. I began to explore the options of scholarship, but this was hard to obtain. I was still optimistic, so I never bothered to think of marriage.

At 27 years of age, an event occurred that warranted an immediate change of plan in finding the appropriate lady to approach for marriage. This involved comments from Donald's wife, Lamin. Lamin's uncle, a pastor, whom Donald respected and adored very much, visited them at their Onitcha residence and was talking to Lamin when I walked in. I greeted the pastor and sat down.

'How are you, Hippo, and what have you been doing since completing your MSc? Do you have any employment yet?' he asked.

'Sort of; I have not gone out in full force in search of a job yet because I am self-employed at the moment, and hope to get foreign admission for my PhD,' I responded with a smile on my face.

'Haven't you studied enough? Don't you know that Donald's children are now beginning to grow up, so he has to save his money for their education too?' retorted the pastor.

I was very embarrassed, and looked down. I wondered what need there was for such a scolding. The next words I heard were the final nail in the coffin. It was Lamin's voice: 'Uncle, the only reason my husband and I are still talking about this is because we need people who will move overseas now so as to use them to move our children over later'.

I was disappointed to hear this selfish grand plan of Lamin and her husband. I resolved right there that I would cancel the idea of travelling if it was only via my brother's sponsorship. I was so disappointed that I wanted to leave immediately. I prayed in my heart before I departed: 'If I ever find the opportunity, I would travel on overseas study but not with my brother's money. Nevertheless, Lord I pray that you so honour me for this insult today so that I could still take at least one of my brother's children overseas to teach them how to be kind in a selfless manner.' What Lamin and her uncle would never have known or imagined was that this prayer was said in my heart right at that spot.

I would have to start thinking of marriage and finally settling down in Nigeria. I decided to relocate to Uyo to live with Papa, operating from there to run my company.

I quietly withdrew from my brother for many years to follow and kept my plans very private. These were the very years when Papa literally invested his life in grooming me, gradually preparing me for a life as a husband and father, teaching me how to become a useful man in society. Papa and his wife would take me along with them to attend occasions, using every opportunity to teach me. It had now been nearly five years on since I relocated to Uyo and I was turning into a real man; hence I sought a wife and got married.

One year after getting married, an opportunity called and I had my chance to go to Royal University London to study for a PhD. But I had no funds to pay for this. I sought financial help from everyone I could think of, including the government of my state of origin and the Federal Ministries of Health, Education, Science and Technology. They all refused me. I contacted relations and friends, but they all failed me.

As described earlier, it was the small achievements I had already made as a medical engineer that led to my opportunity to attend Royal University for six years of full-time education, covering another MSc, PhD degree and two Diplomas from the Royal. No one offered me any financial help, including my brothers and uncles, all through my time in England. One hundred percent credit goes to God, who performed miracles in generating all the required funds through my incessant trips back to Nigeria for work among the hospitals.

I did not bother that no one helped me because I would always remind myself that I was an adult with a wife and a child; hence, it was wrong to think like a child. For lack of funds, my admission was initially deferred for one year before I left for England. Therefore I started to transfer my local monies to my brother Donald's account to enable him to pay the Royal towards my tuition whenever my brother travelled to London; Donald travelled quite often to London for business and also had a London and France bank accounts to save up any balances for me.

I never envisaged the treatment I would later receive from my brother. Donald transferred my money as agreed and using this to part-pay the Royal on one occasion before my arrival in England. The rest of the money was to be transferred to my personal account once I opened it. But it took many calls and much pleading before Donald would transfer my money. He did this in such small quantities that I finally stopped sending my local naira income through my brother.

At the end of my PhD course, I prepared an account statement, with all the Nigerian and London bank cheques, tellers and other documents detailing the transactions between Donald and me. Based on the prevailing money exchange rates at various times of transfer to my brother, the account balances showed that Donald still owed me some money, but I was no longer interested in this unpaid balance. I made copies of the documents and arranged them in duplicate folders.

I gave my brother the honour of being the first person in Nigeria to be notified about the good news of my PhD award in 2006. I was however shocked with the subsequent reaction. The very next day, Donald forwarded a text message he had obviously sent to many relations at home. This read: 'Please help me thank God. After many years of working hard and spending so much money I have finally sponsored my brother Hippolite to obtain his PhD from the prestigious Royal University London'.

I was infuriated by this deceptive message. I was not angry that my brother had failed to transfer all my money or to offer me any financial assistance whatsoever all through the six years of my difficult studentship, but to lie that he had been the one to fund me was like breaking into God's own home and stealing His praise from Him. It was a step too far.

I called Donald and begged him to send a corrective text message to all the people and forwarding the same to me, but Donald refused. I returned to Nigeria during my next hospital consultancy visit, taking the two financial folders I had prepared with me. I went to Donald in the company of my mother and my elder sister and announced that I had important information for all three. Donald had not seen this coming. I began: 'What I am holding here in these folders contains all my financial dealings with my brother since I began my plans for a PhD in London. I hope none of you have been deceived, because I received no iota of financial support from anyone throughout these past six years – brother, sister, uncle, aunt, in-law, name them. I received nothing from anyone, including any of you here listening to me. I don't hold this against anyone because I went to school in London as an adult and should bear the responsibilities between myself and my God. I am also happy today that I achieved my dream through God's special financial miracle. However, my brother Donald has been telling people he sponsored my PhD in London – a terrible lie. I begged him to go round all the people he had deceived to correct his wrong message, but there is no evidence that he did so. Therefore, I need to notify my brother that I have already gone to many of our relations, including his own parents-in-law, those whom he was very likely to have sent the text message, with this file in my hand to show them that my brother actually fabricated a lie to deceive them. In fact, the account balance showed that he still has part of my money, but I don't need this any longer. I want to beg my big brother to stop doing this because it is actually God who you are robbing of His glory'.

I handed Donald one copy of the folders and waited for his response, while the other two watched in amazement and confusion. Donald said nothing. He collected the folder, opened it and read through. He looked up and said: 'Thank you'. I stood and excused myself and left.

After this, I considered my brother unable to manage such vital information without using it selfishly for his own ego, so I decided to stop telling good news first to him. When Donald realised that he was no longer the first to hear any of the subsequent and frequent professional progresses I was making, he began to hate and antagonise me. I was however proud, after a couple of years, to take the opportunity to pick up Donald's daughter and take her to Scotland for a Master's Degree course, completely funded by myself, and afterwards plotted and got her into a very rewarding job with an international health organisation in Nigeria. This fulfilled my prayer the very day I walked out of Donald's house at Onitcha due to the offensive comments from his wife and her uncle.

What next?

I might have thought that I stumbled into the neonatal

challenge by mistake in 1996 at Mbong, or any way it might be defined; however, with what I know today, I would conclude that everything has been divinely orchestrated. When I began, I thought I could solve the entire neonatal mortality problem in Nigeria as one man, but today I know better. I thought that if I could work through all the teaching hospitals and federal medical centres of Nigeria with my ideas, I would defeat the nationally high neonatal mortality rate, but today I know otherwise, because all the tertiary hospitals put together constitute less than 20% of the environs that harbour the needy neonates. The bulk of the cases have remained in the rural areas, the local communities and the hinterlands far away from the city-located tertiary hospitals.

It feels almost hopeless to think that after a quarter of a century of my neonatal adventure, the battle can only be said to have been set under way, not fully won. It has been a gruelling, bumpy, 25-year ride, completely concealed within the hidden places of the tertiary hospitals, catering as they do for less than 20% of these tiny but important lives. The tertiaries seem to have played the role of being the environs for developing and validating the strategies that could guarantee total victory for the neonates. The main battle is about to begin, I suppose.

I and my tiny group would not be the only players. This book has exposed atrocities, in hospitals, in offices, in government, in universities and in high places. This book has conveyed the cries of the babies that were hidden away from the public eye. This book has introduced the topic. So, who would dare to rise up to defend the defenceless? Who still has the mercy to echo and amplify the tiny sound of the crying of these poor neonates? Who still has his conscience intact?

The final battleground is not only at the tertiary hospitals. It is primarily at the community levels where we encounter over 80% of the needy neonates. I invite one and I invite all to come and join hands to save the Nigerian neonate. I have set a new model in place as the final battle-winning strategy. It has been six years since I did this. As usual, the undesirable caterpillars and less-concerned professionals heard me, but looked away. The model is known as the Neonatal Rescue Scheme (NRS). The model would ensure undelayed access to appropriate neonatal intervention, even in the most remote parts of Nigeria. It constitutes 'neonatal hubs' and clusters of 'neorooms'. The Niger State of Nigeria seems to be the only state that has captured the idea, although Yobe state is quietly taking the lead. Yobe is ahead in this race, and if not delayed, it will take Africa by storm by being the first region to reduce neonatal mortality rate to the barest minimum. Having gone up to 70% in readiness to roll out the NRS, my spirit and the spirit of every neonate pray that Yobe state is not held back, so that the rest of Nigeria and Africa may learn from them.

The real hero

It has been a breathtaking, bumpy 25-year ride for me across the jungles, creeks, deserts and cities. I have battled with lay people, nurses, doctors, engineers, civil servants and CMDs who treated the neonates with disrespect – but do not ever think that this makes me the hero. Very recently a CMD complained to me that the frequent breakdown of neonatal devices was a result of the carelessness of his staff team at the SCBU. He complained that these staff do such things without minding how much they are making him suffer as a manager as he continues to worry about the setbacks, or how much I have suffered as I keep coming back to fix these items.

I listened but initially refused to comment. He resumed his complaints before I questioned him: 'Do you suppose that you are the hero, or do you suppose that I am the hero in this whole matter? What pains do we incur to make these fellows pity us and stop the madness? We may complain and worry selfishly – but are we the heroes? We may suffer, but our suffering is nothing compared with that of the neonates that pay the ultimate price of this wickedness with their lives. The neonates are the true heroes!

Statistically, based on the latest demographic report of 2019, in the 24 hours between your breakfast yesterday and today, Nigeria has buried 800 babies, most of which have died from preventable causes. This is like blowing up two jumbo airliners full of babies EVERY DAY. Please do not hide this book and pretend you never read it, because the Nigerian neonate was BORN TO LIVE – NOT TO DIE.

APPENDICES

✦✦✦✦✦✦✦

Appendix 1

Selected public reactions extracted from visitors' register during exhibitions

First ever Nigeria's Technology summit, ABUJA 1997

1. Maj-Gen Sam Momah (*Hon Minister of Science & Technology*)

   "Your products are as good, if not better than imported ones. Please keep it up and be in contact in case of any assistance." (19th May, 1997)

2. Engr (Dr) E J S Uujamhan (*President, Nigerian Society of Engineers*)

   "I found a young establishment fulfilling the vision and mission of the Nigerian Engineer. Remember to always improve every year and you will reach the Summit. I congratulate you to infinity." (19th May, 1997).

3. Dr. Oni Idigbe (*Nigerian Institute of Medical Research, Yaba, Lagos*)

    "Your efforts are encouraging and I will advise you reach out on more research Institutes, private diagnostic laboratories as well as Federal and State health establishments." (22nd May, 1997)

4. Engr (Dr) Charles Uko (*Commissioner for Works, Akwa Ibom State*)

    "Very encouraging work. The finishing standard is highly impressive. There's a lot of prospects for this organization." (20th May, 1997)

5. Prof C O N Wambebe (*Director, NIPRD, Abuja*)

    "Please keep up the excellent effort of designing and fabricating research and hospital equipment." (22nd May, 1997)

6. Dr U S Abdulahi (*Teaching Hospital, ABU, Zaria*)

    "It is impressive to see that these lab equipment are manufactured in Nigeria by Nigerians. Maximum encouragement should be given to the manufacturers to improve and perfect their trade so that foreign exchange can be conserved." (21st May, 1997)

7. Dr V A Fodeke (*FEPA, ABUJA*)

    "WHOW I could not believe it that we have arrived! 100% input for a basic tool for analytical work on. Science, Health and Environment! Good indeed. Great work. Keep it up:" (21st May, 1997)

8. Engr. C C Emekoma (*Chairman, NSE, Owerri Branch*)

    "The products are quite exceptional - with good performance and excellent finish, with excellent prizing that demands encouragement of all. Keep it up." (19th May, 1997)

9. Engr. E. C. Onyeiwu (*Chairman, NSE, Kaduna Branch*)
"Very brilliant contribution to Engineering development". (19th May, 1997)

10. Mr. O. M. Bamson (*Director, Pel-a-Bel Ltd, Abuja*)
"We've seen them in pictures. Now physically. Yes, we've seen them all. Wonderful and unbelievable that they are manufactured in Nigeria. God will prosper your efforts and bring you to highest heights." (21st May, 1997).

Paediatrics Association of Nigeria Conference, PANCONF ILORIN 1998

11. Prof. B. C. Ibe (*Department of Paediatrics, UNTH, Enugu*)
"Very Excellent. Please keep it up" (4th February, 1998)

12. Prof. W. N. Ogala (*ABUTH, Zaria*)
"Very impressive" (4th February, 1998)

At other times

13. Nigerian Engineers led by Engr. C. A. Mbanefo (*President of the Nigerian Society of Engineers*)

"This visit is an eye opener. The achievement of this centre is a good testimony to what Nigerian Engineers can do, given the vital support. There should be a presentation of the equipment to the Nation" (inspection of developed neonatal systems 1999)

14. Paediatric Doctors led by Prof. J. C. Azubuike (*Head of Paediatrics Department, UNTH, Enugu, and Chairman of Paediatrics, National Postgraduate Medical College of Nigeria*)

"I remain impressed by the products of your company. I am happy to confirm that my initial impressions of Engineer H. Amadi remain unchanged. Please keep it up." (inspection of developed neonatal systems, 1999)

Appendix 2

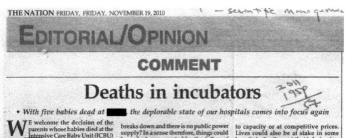

THE NATION FRIDAY, FRIDAY, NOVEMBER 19, 2010

EDITORIAL/OPINION

COMMENT

Deaths in incubators

- With five babies dead at ███, the deplorable state of our hospitals comes into focus again

WE welcome the decision of the parents whose babies died at the Intensive Care Baby Unit (ICBU) of the ███versity Teaching Hospital ███ State, to sue the hospital's management. According to the parents, the babies died as a result of power failure that lasted over two hours.

The hospital's authorities have however denied that the babies died due to power failure since there is a stand-by generator that comes up immediately power goes off. Indeed, a doctor in the hospital claimed that the babies died either of congenital infections or because they were born pre-term, and not because of power failure.

For now, it is the words of the hospital's management against those of the bereaved parents, and an investigation might have to be carried out to know the ████ of the ██████ death. But

breaks down and there is no public power supply? In a sense therefore, things could be as bad as presented by the father of one of the dead babies, ████, to the effect that he sometimes went to the hospital with his lantern, to assist the doctors who sometimes work with torch lights.

This scenario presents us with two problems: power supply and the deplorable state of health facilities in the country. In other words, ███ is only a metaphor for the deplorable state of our medical institutions. Yet, it is supposed to be 'Centre of excellence for gastro intestinal disease'. Most of our hospitals, including the so-called teaching hospitals, are only shadows of what they were in the 1970s and '80s. They do not have the basic equipment that are taken for granted in hospitals which in no way come near being 'cen-

to capacity or at competitive prices. Lives could also be at stake in some hospitals. So, the cost that is being imputed for power problems is far beyond the ones we could denominate in naira and kobo. So, we have to fix the power problem and many other things will naturally follow.

In like manner, our hospitals do not need high-sounding names to be effective and efficient. Rather, they need the best of working tools that we can afford. Most of the rich people in the country often travel abroad for routine medical check-ups. If we compute what these cost us in foreign exchange, we would be astonished. We should always bear in mind that if the people in other countries where our rich flock to over minor ailments did nothing to improve healthcare in their countries, our influ-

Appendix 3
My research coverage by Nigerian states

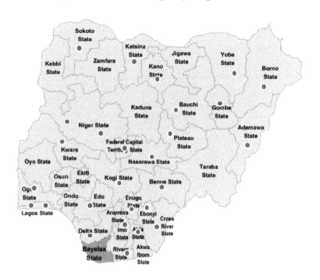

Appendix 4
Daily newborn mortality 2007-2018 in Nigeria

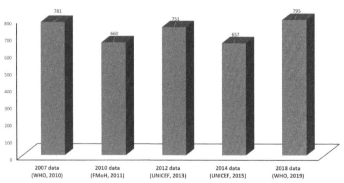

Described as crashing TWO JUMBO JETS OF BABIES every day in Nigeria, UNICEF Kaduna, 2019

ND - #0245 - 270225 - C0 - 203/127/25 - PB - 9781861519528 - Gloss Lamination